Praise for *Thriving*

"Dr. Sotile is, without question, this country's leading authority on the psychological, emotional, and relationship effects of making it through heart disease. His understanding and compassion will be invaluable for heart patients who are coping with and living through the initial diagnosis and treatment of the illness, and then living the rest of their lives with it. For patients with heart disease and those who care about and for them, this book is a must-read."

—Harry Croft, M.D., medical director and founder
of the San Antonio Psychiatric Research Center

"Dr. Sotile is one of the world's brightest psychologists. Dr. Sotile's advice will help all individuals with cardiovascular disease, as well as those who are at risk of developing heart disease."

—Gordon A. Ewy, M.D., professor and chief cardiology
director, University of Arizona Sarver Heart Center

"This wonderful book fills a critical void for patients by dealing with the day-to-day emotional and psychosocial challenges of heart disease—managing stress, managing anger and hostility, dealing with depression, and resuming sexual activity. [I]t answers many important questions that are seldom if ever addressed by physicians and health care providers."

—Barry A. Franklin, Ph.D., director, Cardiac Rehabilitation
and Exercise Laboratories, William Beaumont Hospital,
coauthor of *Take a Load Off Your Heart*

"Dr. Sotile has made a significant contribution to the understanding of heart health. Comprehensive and cutting-edge, it's required reading for heart patients and their families. I highly recommend it."

—Joseph C. Piscatella, coauthor of *Take a Load Off Your Heart*

"*Thriving with Heart Disease* is far more than a self-help book. Educational, informational, and compassionate, it offers guidance and reassurance to cardiac patients and their families to enhance their recovery. Particularly welcome is its attention to women as heart patients, a topic commonly neglected in other presentations."

—Nanette K. Wenger, M.D., professor of medicine, Emory University School of Medicine, and chief of cardiology, Grady Memorial Hospital

"[A] gift to anyone with heart disease. Coping with the emotional stress of a life-threatening illness is a major challenge, and Dr. Sotile's insights, warmth, and empathy—combined with sound advice—will improve every reader's quality of life. This book should be read by anyone touched by heart disease: patients, their families, and their friends. Everyone will benefit."

—Kathy Berra, M.S.N., N.P., F.A.A.N.

"This is a wonderful guide—loving, practical, straight-talking, uplifting, and helpful. Reading it, you feel as if Dr. Sotile is your best friend, that he's got the answer to every question that's worrying you, and that nothing is too small or insignificant to ask about. . . . It's magic."

—Diane Sollee, founder and director, Coalition for Marriage, Family, and Couples Education; and *www.smartmarriages.com*

Other Books by Wayne M. Sotile, Ph.D.

PSYCHOSOCIAL INTERVENTIONS
FOR CARDIOPULMONARY PATIENTS

THE MEDICAL MARRIAGE

Sustaining Healthy Relationships
for Physicians and Their Families
(cowritten with Mary O. Sotile, M.A.)

THE RESILIENT PHYSICIAN

Effective Emotional Management for Doctors
and Their Medical Organizations
(cowritten with Mary O. Sotile, M.A.)

MARRIAGE SKILLS FOR BUSY COUPLES

How to Avoid Supercouple Syndrome
(cowritten with Mary O. Sotile, M.A.)

THRIVING WITH HEART DISEASE

*The Leading Authority on the Emotional
Effects of Heart Disease Tells You and Your
Family How to Heal and Reclaim Your Lives*

❖

Wayne M. Sotile, Ph.D.,
with Robin Cantor-Cooke

FREE PRESS
New York   London   Toronto   Sydney

To the heroic heart patients at the
Wake Forest University Cardiac Rehabilitation Program:
You teach us all lessons about living.

*f*P

FREE PRESS
A Division of Simon & Schuster, Inc.
1230 Avenue of the Americas
New York, NY 10020

First Free Press trade paperback edition 2004

FREE PRESS and colophon are trademarks
of Simon & Schuster, Inc.

For information about special discounts for bulk purchases,
please contact Simon & Schuster Special Sales:
1-800-456-6798 or business@simonandschuster.com

Designed by Lisa Chovnick

Manufactured in the United States of America

3   5   7   9   10   8   6   4

Library of Congress Cataloging-in-Publication Data
Sotile, Wayne M., 1951–
Thriving with heart disease : a unique program for you and your family : live happier,
healthier, longer / Wayne M. Sotile, with Robin Cantor-Cooke.
p. cm.
1. Heart—Diseases—Psychological aspects—Popular works.   I. Cantor-Cooke, Robin.
II. Title.

RC682.S643   2003   362.1'9612—dc21   2002045587

ISBN 978-0-7432-4365-0
ISBN 074324365X

Permissions appear on pages 302–3.

ACKNOWLEDGMENTS

I thank the many people who help me thrive:

My esteemed colleagues and valued friends at the Wake Forest University Cardiac Rehabilitation Program—pioneers, one and all, but, more important, nice people.

Kathy Hall—for living up to the recommendation offered by your prior employer: "The minute you hire this woman, your life will be at least fifty percent better than it was the minute before."

My great staff and colleagues at Sotile Psychological Associates—for making ours the best and most pleasant practice anyone ever called home.

My agent, Gail Ross—for your astute guidance in shaping this project, your amazing business savvy and professionalism, and believing in me long before this book was born.

The visionary folks at Free Press—for your enthusiasm and passion about this book and me. Special thanks to Philip Rappaport for convincing me, and to Leslie Meredith for guiding me, and to Dorothy Robinson for your gracious and tireless support and attention to the details that brought us to completion.

Lynn Anderson—for your superb copyediting and devotion to detail.

Samuel F. Sears, Ph.D.—for your collaboration, collegiality, and friendship; and for your own pioneering work in cardiac psychology.

Barbara H. Ballow Lankton, M.D.—for your helpful comments and guidance regarding medications, and for being an enduring island of safety for so many of our shared patients.

Steven Ackerman, M.D.—for educating me about cutting-edge cardiac technologies.

Rochelle Kramer—for your invaluable and gracious assistance with library searches.

The many hospitals, pharmaceutical companies, and medical technology companies—for continuing to sponsor educational events that help heart patients and their families.

The American Association of Cardiovascular and Pulmonary Rehabilitation and its many state affiliates—for providing us all with forums in which we can teach and support one another.

James A. Blumenthal, Ph.D.; Redford Williams, M.D.; Margaret Chesney, Ph.D.; Robert Allan, Ph.D.; Karen Matthews, Ph.D.; Lynda H. Powell, Ph.D.; Diane K. Ulmer, R.N., M.S.; Kathleen Dracup, D.N.Sc., R.N.; and many others—for blazing the trail into cardiac psychology.

The leadership of the American Psychological Association—for continuing to underscore the importance of incorporating psychological care into cardiac care.

My valued friends and colleagues from the American College of Cardiology—Robert Superko, M.D.; Hugh Smith, M.D.; Timothy Fleming, M.D.; and Meredith L. Scott, M.D.—for doing so much to help so many physicians to better care for heart patients, and for allowing me to participate in your efforts.

Robin Cantor-Cooke—for your infectious enthusiasm, gracious collaboration, and stellar writing. You make my ideas sing!

My daughters, Rebecca and Julia—for keeping my heart open. And my wife and only partner, Mary—for making my dreams come true. I love each of you with my life.

CONTENTS

PREFACE

Since the hardcover edition of *Thriving with Heart Disease* was released a year ago, I have been warmed by gratitude that has poured forth from heart patients and their families. Their enthusiasm for the book has affirmed my purpose in writing it: to give heart patients and the people who love them information they need and crave on coping with the psychological challenges of the disease.

This volume, the first paperback edition, contains all the content from the hardcover plus a little bit more. I can describe the new material best by digging down to my south Louisiana roots and pulling up a Cajun tradition called "lagniappe," which sounds like "lan-yap" and is something you get as a bonus—usually an unexpected, savory tidbit from the chef to persuade you to return to the restaurant. This volume contains a nourishing portion of lagniappe: updates on women and heart illness, advice for adults who are shocked to learn they've been walking around with a heart abnormality all their lives, new angles on how to manage relationships with your doctors, and more.

I hope these updates inspire you to return to this book time and again for guidance and encouragement. I also hope you will write to me or visit my Web site, www.thrivingwithheartdisease.com, and tell me your story. Many readers have opened their hearts and told me about their journeys and in so doing have enriched me beyond measure. They have my constant gratitude and admiration.

Wayne M. Sotile
Winston-Salem, North Carolina

FOREWORD

In the last decade of the twentieth century, medical science made tremendous advances in the diagnosis, treatment, and prevention of heart disease. Physicians now have procedures that open blocked arteries (angioplasty) and reroute clogged plumbing (coronary artery bypass surgery). We use medicines that dissolve arterial clots that cause heart attacks. We also have "magic pills"—medications that increase patients' chances of survival: statins that lower cholesterol, ACE inhibitors for blood pressure, aspirin to prevent blood clotting. And the list is growing.

These medications save lives, and the procedures are improving so patients can leave the hospital and go home faster. But faster does not always mean better. Nor does it mean that the patients are emotionally ready to go home. Physicians and hospitals—or, rather, their insurance companies—now send people home within five days of their heart attacks and heart surgery.

Yet research consistently shows that even when heart surgeries and other treatments are technically successful, the men and women who have undergone them don't always return to their normal lives. That's because heart health requires more than a "golden cholesterol level" or eating five servings of fruit and vegetables each day. How you *feel* about your heart disease, the stressors that act upon you at home and on the job, *all* affect your heart's health. If you feel your head pounding or face reddening during the weekday commute, you may find yourself back in the emergency room, despite the fact that your operation was a success and your medications are helping you stay physically healthy.

Your mind is an important player in your heart disease, and the evidence for a mind-body connection is compelling. If you tend to get angry, if you have little control over your work environment, if you are isolated from your friends and family, or if you are depressed about your illness, you will damage your heart. Stress and anger have real effects on the heart and blood vessels. As you sit in traffic thinking about being late for a meeting, for instance, your stress hormones jump into action. Adrenaline and cortisol surge and your heart rate and blood pressure increase, potentially causing direct damage to your blood vessels.

For total heart health, you need a healthy mind. You've survived your heart attack or hypertension. You're eating a healthier diet. You're taking your medications. Now it's time for you to take care of *your whole self.* It's time for you to tend to your emotions and improve your life. As I tell my patients, life-saving therapies assure you of a longer life, but now it's time to *get* a life. *Thriving with Heart Disease* will help you. It is the next step in your recovery. Dr. Sotile shows you how to deal with emotions and stresses that you may not even have been conscious you had but that have nonetheless been keeping you from being fully well.

While doctors in general and cardiologists specifically are getting better at addressing obvious heart disease risk factors such as high blood pressure, diabetes, high cholesterol, smoking, and lack of exercise, they are not necessarily paying closer attention to the very real emotions such as depression, anger, and stress that accompany the disease. These factors have been proven to put people at risk for developing heart disease and prevent patients from having a better quality of life after a heart attack or heart surgery. If these factors are left untreated, they can increase the risk for worsening heart disease or more heart attacks. If you're a heart patient, dealing with your fears, anxieties, and emotions is key to your full recovery. *Thriving with Heart Disease* can help you do all this and get yourself a better, healthier life than before.

Every morning, I see a photograph of one of my patients on my bookcase. Gregory is standing with his wife and four-year-old daughter after having run a race. What makes this picture different is that seven months before it was taken, Gregory, then fifty-four years old, had had a major heart attack. His photo represents the importance of the mind in healing the heart. Gregory, like many men who have had heart attacks, had a driven personality. A time-pressured, competitive, and hostile stockbroker, he was rude on the phone when he scheduled his initial visit to our cardiac rehabilitation program. In fact, our physical therapist told me she was tempted to recommend him to another program. I pointed out, however, that his hostility was one of the reasons he had had a heart attack and needed our help. After we gave Gregory an appointment, he changed it six times, insisting that we change our schedule to accommodate his, a common problem with hard-driving personalities. After some negotiation, he joined our program.

During my conversations with Gregory, he admitted that he was angry about his heart attack, as many patients are; he had been physically active and had exercised all his life, including running in the New York City Marathon, yet he had had a heart attack. He was also worried because he had married late in life and feared he would no longer be able to take care of his family or live to see his daughter go to college. Gregory also wanted to run a marathon again.

I told Gregory that his heart attack was his second chance at life. For him, the exercise portion of recovery would be easy, but if he were to heal completely and not have to worry about suffering another heart attack, he also would have to work on how he handled his emotions, especially his anger and constant sense of urgency. I also explained that he would not be able to change everything overnight. We organized a plan, he faithfully attended the stress management sessions at the program, and set sensible goals for himself. For instance, instead of training for the New York City Marathon, he participated in shorter runs for a couple of months.

Gregory was also very worried about his wife's intimacy problems. This is an almost universal concern of heart patients and their spouses and partners. Gregory felt like a failure because every time he wanted to have sex or discuss sex with his wife, she pulled away. Thankfully, she agreed to meet with him and me and was able to admit that she was terribly anxious that Gregory would have another heart attack if they made love. After I reassured them that his medical condition did not indicate a probable second heart attack, they decided to seek counseling and eventually resumed their love life.

With a combination of medication, exercise, emotion management, and his family's help, Gregory's entire life improved. He said it was even better than before his heart attack. Gregory's story shows why it is important to heal the mind as well as the body. The best medications and medical treatments alone would not have put him back together. He, like so many other men and women, needed the support of his family, plus counseling to help him modify his responses to strong emotions and to reorganize his life. Without this mind-body approach to his cardiac rehabilitation, he may well have found himself back in the emergency room. Gregory is a success not just because he actually ran the Marathon, but because he was able to break the cycle of his heart-attack-prone behavior.

Depression, stress, and heart-attack-prone behavior are not exclusive to men. Women also experience these risk factors for heart disease. Their lives and symptoms, however, often differ from those of men. Jessica was only thirty-eight when she had her heart attack. She doesn't remember much about it because she was brought to the hospital unconscious: Her first symptom was cardiac arrest. She actually died and was brought back to life. Even though Jessica had had the heart attack three years before she saw me, she could not stop thinking about it. She obsessively reviewed a cycle of questions: How did it happen? Would it happen again? She sometimes had chest pain and palpitations and wondered if she would faint again, as she had during the heart attack. She would rarely go out, was too frightened to exercise, and felt alienated from her husband and children, who, she said, didn't know what to say to her.

Jessica was having a very hard time trying to get over her fears about the heart attack and the possibility of future ones. She felt as though she had no control over her health. Yet Jessica had received excellent care; during her hospitalization, an angiogram revealed an artery blockage that her doctors subsequently cleared. They told her she was "fixed"; but, while the physical problem in her artery was healed, Jessica wasn't.

Because women often repress their anger, they may not be as outwardly hostile as men, but anger—whether or not you express it—takes its toll on the heart. Women also suffer from depression twice as often as do men, which reduces their ability to survive heart disease. When I began working with Jessica, she had withdrawn from her friends and felt she would have another heart attack if she exerted herself to do laundry or straightened the bed in the morning. She was angry at her family because she mistakenly felt that they didn't care enough about her and were not helping her enough, yet she kept this anger and resentment to herself. Before she began to tell her family about her fears and her need for help, Jessica was a perfect example of a woman who had survived a serious heart attack, yet was not thriving with her heart disease. Once her family realized how scared she was, and once Jessica began to confront her fears and see for herself that she was *physically* healed, she began to live her life again.

Recovering from heart disease takes time. After all, it took many years for your arteries to become clogged—years of no exercise, or of eating foods high in fat, or of smoking. If you constantly felt pressured, angry, or depressed, the physical effects of these emotions also contributed to your heart disease. Your survival and your health are certainly improved by high-tech procedures and medications, but if you neglect your emotional well-being, you will *not* heal completely. Your goal is not merely to *survive* your heart disease; it is to *thrive with* it. Dr. Sotile's program in *Thriving with Heart Disease* can be the most important step of your life toward complete emotional and heart health.

—Nieca Goldberg, M.D.,
Chief, Women's Heart Program,
Lenox Hill Hospital (New York City, NY);
Member of the American Heart
Association National Spokesperson's Panel;
and author of *Women Are Not Small Men*

PART ONE

❖

CONGRATULATIONS ON YOUR HEART ILLNESS—YOU GOT A SECOND CHANCE!

Chapter One

BEGIN THE JOURNEY

I am a cardiac psychologist. For nearly twenty-five years I have been helping people recover from heart disease by teaching them and their loved ones how to contend with the emotional ravages of the illness. This book is the fruit of countless hours I've spent with thousands of heart patients and their families—men and women like you, with loved ones like yours. My message will knock your life back onto its feet because I'm going to tell you something about heart disease you may not have known before: it's not the severity of the illness but how you cope with it that will determine how long you will live and how happy you will be.[1] *Not only can you survive heart disease, you can actually thrive with it for many, many years.* In fact, if you cope well and follow the advice I give you in this book, you can live as long as you would if you didn't have the illness.

That's right: you can live as long as you would if you didn't have the illness. And you can lead a full and vibrant life, a life of challenge and discovery. You don't have to live like an invalid, propped up in a corner of the couch while your days diminish into a series of bland, limited routines. You don't have to tiptoe through your nights and days, anxious that a backfiring truck or a spin on the dance floor will throw you into the hospital with a heart attack. And you don't have to suffer from New Age guilt because you couldn't swallow the diet of the month or stick with the latest exercise fad.

What you *do* have to do is acknowledge the gift you've received: the infinite bounty of a second chance. The fact that you are holding this book and reading these words confirms your place among the privileged, the lucky ones who got the wake-up call, resisted the urge to slam the snooze button, and chose to embark on the journey toward a newly conscious life. Because living with heart disease *is* a journey—a journey forward toward the healthy life you were meant to live, not back to the one you were living when the illness struck. It's a journey you take one moment at a time— breakfast by breakfast and conversation by conversation, embrace by embrace and, yes, conflict by conflict. It's a journey you'll be taking for the rest of your life—which, I remind you, can be a long, long time—and the people who love you the most get to come with you.

That's the thing that astonishes so many of my patients: the degree to which their illness is a family affair. Heart disease can cause a seismic shift in even the most stable relationships, rattling a family's foundation and leaving its members shaky and grim. It's always unsettling but worst when the illness strikes without warning, which happens more often than you might think: *All known cardiac risk factors combined account for only three out of four cases of heart illness*—the others are attributed to unknown causes.

There are also millions of people living with cardiac complications due to congenital heart defects. When these defects are diagnosed at birth or during childhood, the people who have them grow up knowing about the condition (and, in the best-case scenarios, managing it). There are even cases in which a doctor discovers a heart defect in a developing fetus and operates on the baby in utero, correcting the problem before the child is born. But in other cases a problem can go undetected until one day a person visits the doctor and finds out that he or she has been walking around with a heart abnormality for fifty years—at best a surprising event and sometimes a shocking and disorienting one, especially when it happens later in life.[2]

If you are like most heart patients, your notion of normal changed forever the instant you were diagnosed with heart disease or a congenital heart defect. Suddenly, nothing was the same for you or your family, and everything ended in a question mark:

- Am I going to die?
- Why did this happen to me?
- What happens now?
- How will we manage?
- Will things ever be the same?

You all probably have had to deal with unfamiliar people (doctors, nurses, rehabilitation specialists, technicians), unfamiliar places (hospitals, waiting rooms), and unpleasant experiences (procedures, tests, surgery). How you manage these experiences—as a patient and as a family—will determine the quality of your life and how long you hold on to it. Thriving with heart disease isn't only about a muscle, it's also about how you manage your emotions, your attitude, and the intricate web of human connections, secure and tenuous, that bind you to the people you love and interact with.

And thriving doesn't stop with family relationships: *the way a patient interacts with others can determine how long and happily he or she will live.* A married loner with no close friends, few acquaintances, and a not-very-serious heart condition may never recover fully, while a quiet person who lives alone but has vibrant friendships and cordial family relations may resume an active life even after a whopper of a heart attack.

That's what pulled Rena and Tom through: strong family relations. The topography of their marriage had changed forever three years earlier, when Rena suffered a myocardial infarction, or heart attack.*

Tom stands well over six feet tall, weighs about 230 pounds, and has one of those steel gray crew cuts that makes some men look like unusually mature marines. They had come to my office to talk about how they as a couple were living with heart disease. As Tom rose from the waiting room chair, he offered a large, open hand to Rena. I was struck by her presence; her handshake was as firm as her gaze. Tom spoke first:

"It was simple: I knew Rena was going to die. I was so frightened of losing her, I didn't even allow myself to think she might pull through. I just wanted to try to prepare myself for the worst, so if it happened, it wouldn't be a complete shock.

"In the hospital, I just waited and waited for her to open her eyes. I kept wondering, why did this happen? Rena's family didn't have heart problems. I thought it must be a mistake, that they'd made the wrong diagnosis. The kids came every day, they took off from work . . . we surrounded each other with love; that's how we got through.

"Rena made it over the first hurdle—she got out of the hospital. Then we had another surprise—coming home. Boy, those first few months were a shock. At first I tried to do everything—the cooking, the laundry, the marketing, everything. Then, later on, I slowly let her take over, little by little."

Now Rena looked up and began to speak:

"The first six months were the worst. Some mornings I'd wake up not caring about anything. One day, I didn't even fix my hair. I remember thinking I must be losing my grip; I'd always paid attention to my appearance. But I figured, what's the difference? I wasn't going anywhere, no one was going to see me except Tom.

---

* I have changed the names of my patients to preserve their privacy; some case histories are composites of several patients.

"I also worried that I couldn't rely on my body anymore. One day I needed a blanket up in the linen closet, and I was afraid to get up on a step stool to get it down. I thought I'd lose my balance and fall—off a step stool, for goodness' sake! So I sat down on the floor and cried for half an hour.

"And then there were the panic attacks. Whenever something felt different in my chest area I immediately thought, oh, no, something's happening—another artery is blocking up, and I'm going to end up in an ambulance. For a few months, I was a nervous wreck.

"Tom and the kids were very worried about me. They didn't let me do anything, even things I wanted to do. One Sunday I got it in my head I wanted to clean out the pantry. It was the first time in weeks I'd felt like doing anything, and it made me happy. The kids were over that day, and, well, they wouldn't let me do it. The more I insisted, the more they fought me. I finally gave up and went to lie down, and Tom and the kids cleaned out the pantry. It took me three weeks to find the oregano because they put stuff back in the wrong place.

"Here they were, trying to spare me from stress and causing me so much aggravation I had to go lie down. I loved them for all they were doing, but I knew I could do more than they thought I could—especially everyday, normal things."

As Rena and Tom learned, the future is seldom determined at the hospital. The vast majority of heart patients' futures develop gradually, like photographs in processing solution, as they return home and get back to normal—a normal that may be a far cry from what they knew before. And that's precisely the point: when heart illness strikes, a person must abandon the well-trodden path he or she used to follow, blaze a trail, and begin a journey toward a new way of living. Heart disease is an invitation to create a different way of life—a new normal—that heals the heart by tending emotions and mending human connections.

As Tom put it, "We've been married for over forty-two years. We've grown up a lot in that time, and we're still growing. Living with this illness has taught us to keep things in perspective, to be more flexible, and to pay attention to each day we have together. When you do that, life gets better. You know how, early in marriage, sex is such a big deal? I still love sex; it's great. But intimacy is greater."

STARTING THE JOURNEY

Living long and well with heart disease is like driving cross-country to get home for Thanksgiving: it's a long haul, but the party will be a lot better if you're part of it (also, once you're on the road, you'll realize you're not the only one out there). You'll have long stretches where you fly along, making great progress, but you'll also hit detours and obstacles that make you wonder if you'll ever arrive.

I promise: you can and *will* arrive if you follow the program in this book, which places in your hands the same tools and techniques my patients receive at the Wake Forest University Cardiac Rehabilitation Program. Your program starts now, as you open your mind and embrace two fundamental truths: first, that recovery is a journey you'll be taking for the rest of your life, not a signpost you rolled past when you left the hospital. And second, that heart illness will challenge you and the people close to you to open yourselves to one another as never before—even when you feel incapable of a civil "good morning"—and you must rise to the challenge and do it.

I *know* you can do it because I've watched others do it time and time again. Heart patients are my life's work, and this book is the crystallization of my commitment to you, your family, and your future. For many years I have wished I could hand my patients a talisman, a potent object that would keep them from harm and protect them from despair. This book is that talisman, a gift of hope to help you and your family defy the demons of heart illness and win.

Chapter Two

THE FOUR STAGES
OF HEART ILLNESS

As heart patients recover, they pass through a series of separate, identifiable stages. The stages don't always proceed neatly in sequence, but your recovery will have fewer surprises if you are familiar with them and know what to expect.

Here is how the stages progress for most patients and their families:

- **Stage I: Surviving the crisis.** Illness strikes and patient and family begin the journey.
- **Stage II: Creating a coping strategy.** Everyone starts to grasp what heart illness is, what's involved in treatment and recovery, and that the patient and family must work as a team.
- **Stage III: Handling the homecoming blues.** You're suddenly on your own; reality sets in and the team must adapt to its new normal.
- **Stage IV: Learning to live with heart disease.** Patient and family have accepted the diagnosis and committed themselves to living *with* the illness, not in spite of it.

Let's explore the stages one by one.

STAGE I: SURVIVING THE CRISIS

Each patient gets the news in a different way: One may be sitting in her doctor's office, stunned by some test results she hadn't given much thought to; another may land in the emergency room feeling as if a five-hundred-pound gorilla is sitting on his chest. However the news arrives, it hurls you into strange, forbidding territory, and your journey begins.

When the crisis hits, most heart patients and their families put their lives on hold, band together, and try to help one another endure. Petty conflicts are swept aside by a wave of concern for the patient and fear that he or she may not survive. Family members summon reserves of emotional fortitude and reinforce one another with love.

If you're the patient, this wait-and-see period feels as if your future has been torn from your hands and become the property of medical professionals. It's also a time when feelings of helplessness can overwhelm you. You may no longer trust your suddenly unreliable body. Family members also feel helpless as they stand by, waiting for information, hunched with worry.

In the midst of all this vulnerability, it's common for patients and their families to relinquish their autonomy and entrust themselves completely to the physicians and hospital staff. While it's important to trust the people taking care of you, it's also crucial that you maintain your authority and see to it that you're treated as a whole human being and not a set of symptoms. As I've mentioned, thriving with heart disease involves both muscle and mind, and all too often, the psychological aspect of healing is overlooked. There are even some cardiologists who dismiss the notion that mending the mind can help heal the heart. This is why you must see yourself as your physicians' partner, not their child. In the words of Melvin Belsky, M.D., "It's not enough for the doctor to stop playing God—you've got to get off your knees."

The big story here is not only that assertive patients and family members get better care from physicians, but that heart patients *must* be assertive to get the care they need. It's not enough to show up at the doctor's office or emergency room; that's no guarantee you'll be properly cared for. You must hold fast to your independence, trust your instincts, and assert your right to be treated well—both medically and personally.

This means having the confidence to ask a physician to explain what he or she is saying, ordering, or prescribing, and also to express your wishes. This could involve telling your cardiologist that you would like him or her to coordinate your care with your family doctor. A recent Harvard study followed 35,000 heart attack patients for two years after their release from the hospital and found that those who received care from both a cardiologist and a general practitioner had the highest survival rates.[1] Or you might have to assert your right to be treated with dignity: if you feel a physician (or anyone else, for that matter) has been rude or disrespectful or that his or her personality displays an arrogance that is compromising the quality of your care, don't put up with it. Let people know how you would prefer to be treated.

Even something as common as being called by your first name when you'd prefer a less familiar form of address is worth dealing with. Young

---

EXPERIENCE MATTERS!

If you've survived a myocardial infarction (MI, or heart attack) and have a doctor who treats a high volume of MI patients, you are more likely to be alive a year later; a 2001 study found a significant difference in survival rates for patients treated by physicians who treat more than twenty-four MI patients per year versus physicians who treat fewer than five.[2] The same applies if you are undergoing an invasive procedure such as angioplasty: having a physician who frequently performs the surgery and using a hospital where many are done increases your odds of survival.[3] Not surprisingly, the same holds true with more complex cardiac surgery: hospitals with busy operating rooms have lower death rates than hospitals whose ORs sit idle much of the time.[4] It makes good, common sense: the more operations surgeons do, the better they get at it and the better support staff gets at providing high-quality postoperative care.

---

professionals grew up in informal times, calling teachers and sometimes even parents by their first names. When they don their medical coats, they don't always make the leap to those more traditional shores where many of their older patients stand. If it irks you to address thirty-five-year-old physicians as "Doctor" while they assume they may call you by your first name, let them know how you'd like them to address you.

No matter how well you get along with your doctors, however, you'll still have emotions to deal with. Immediately after learning the diagnosis, patients and their families may struggle with bouts of guilt and anxiety. These feelings pervade conversations and thought patterns, taking standard forms such as:

PATIENT: I should have taken better care of myself.

FAMILY MEMBER: I should have been at you more to go to the doctor.

PATIENT: After all we've been through, now this! I can't believe I let this happen.

FAMILY MEMBER: You'd think I'd have been able to see this coming and stop it from happening.

PATIENT: I'll never be the person I was before this happened . . . how will I ever make it up to you?

FAMILY MEMBER: If I'd been a better mate and paid more attention, this would never have happened.

PATIENT: If only I'd been easier to get along with, maybe this wouldn't have happened.

FAMILY MEMBER: If only I'd kept my mouth shut and not given you a hard time last week [last month, last year, five years ago], maybe this wouldn't have happened.

PATIENT: If I die, what will happen to my family?

FAMILY MEMBER: What will we do if something happens? How will we cope?

If your family is emotionally healthy, you should be able to express these feelings, however awkwardly, and then respond to one another with love and concern. But even if your family is emotionally well adjusted, tensions will mount during this early stage. For many people, this stage means coping with being inside a hospital. This can be physically and emotionally (not to mention financially) draining for patients and family members alike. Monitors beep, screens flash, tubes emerge from and disappear into the body. Coolly competent doctors and nurses take charge of the patient, separating him or her from family members, whose warmth and concern are left behind in the corridor. If the patient needs surgery, there is the horror of seeing him or her attached to a respirator. The patient is sedated, cannot speak, and may float into and out of awareness, unable to communicate. For loved ones clustered nearby, the image of the person they love lying pale and helpless may haunt them for the rest of their lives.

While many heart patients have similar experiences in the hospital, their responses—and their families'—vary widely. Many patients take comfort in religion, which seems to heal bodies as well as souls: people over the age of fifty-five who are facing open-heart surgery and are also committed to some form of religious practice have survival rates that are *three times higher* than their nonreligious brothers and sisters.[5]

"WHAT'S THE BIG DEAL? NOTHING'S WRONG WITH ME."

Other patients seem to benefit from denial, a psychological defense that allows them to avoid dealing with the fact that they have heart disease. If you used this technique while you were in the hospital you may have done yourself a favor, as long as it didn't keep you from accepting the medical care you needed. In fact, during the first days of hospitalization, patients who show high levels of denial actually tend to do *better:* they are less anxious, less depressed, and leave the hospital sooner because they have fewer medical complications.[6]

Denial of cardiac illness is a complex issue. One study followed thirty men for a year after their heart attacks, measuring how much they either accepted or denied their condition. The results were fascinating: the most vehement deniers spent fewer days in intensive care and had fewer adjustment struggles while they were in the hospital compared to their more accepting brothers. But once they left the hospital, things changed: one year after their heart attacks, the deniers were less likely to follow their doctors' recommendations, and were landing back in the hospital more than the more accepting patients.[7]

So deniers, take note: while you might benefit from denial during your first days in the hospital, don't take this technique home with you. *Your successful recovery and long-term adjustment require that you accept that you have heart illness and cope with the feelings that come with it.*[8] In most cases this happens naturally; most heart patients start experiencing anxiety and depression after several days in the hospital, which signals that denial is diminishing. If this has happened to you or is happening now, take heart: while these emotions may be painful, they are not dangerous, and they typically decrease with time. If they don't, you can learn to manage anxiety, and you can overcome depression. These conditions are virtually curable with therapy, medication, or a combination of both. You can start treating your anxiety and depression right now by doing two things:

1. **Identify what you are feeling.** It's not enough to say that you've lost your appetite or you don't want to go for a walk, thank you very much— these are verbal manifestations of denial. If you've had more butterflies in your stomach than food lately, quiet your mind until you see them for what they are: anxiety with wings. If you haven't got the energy to launch yourself off the couch and out the door, look inward and ask yourself if it could be depression, and not your legs, that's making you weak.

2. **Tell someone about it.** Once you have got a name for the problem, tell someone about it—your mate, a friend, a daughter or son, a doctor or nurse. Pick a sympathetic listener, someone you trust. If your emotions threaten to get the better of you, take a deep breath and do your best to express yourself calmly and politely. Once you do this, you'll have taken a giant step in your journey toward recovery and the truth.

Some people get stuck in denial mode past when it's beneficial to be there. If you've known for more than a month that you have heart illness and are experiencing any of the following symptoms, you may be at risk of not taking the illness seriously enough. Are you:

- Clinging to the belief that the illness isn't serious when medical evidence suggests that it is?

- Choosing to interpret symptoms of heart illness as those of minor physical ailments (for example, insisting that the crushing pain in your chest is "just gas")?

- Refusing to believe that you're sick in the first place?

- Denying that you need to be admitted to the hospital, and resisting your doctor's and family's attempts to get you there?

- Denying that the illness is going to affect your life or the lives of the people you care about?

WOMEN AND DENIAL

Two excellent books—*The Women's Heart Book*, by Fredric J. Pashkow, M.D., and Charlotte Libov; and *Women Are Not Small Men*, by Nieca Goldberg, M.D.—call attention to a lethal problem: denial that heart illness is a menace to women's health. Our culture still embraces the myth that women don't have to worry about heart illness, but they do: *cardiovascular disease kills more American women each year than breast cancer, lung cancer, and colon cancer combined.*[9]

While women are more likely than men to seek medical care when they think they need it,[10] they seldom think they need it when it comes to their hearts. When women suffer heart attack symptoms, they tend to misattribute their symptoms to noncardiac causes,[11] waiting longer than men do to seek medical help.

There also seem to be differences in the ways black women experience symptoms compared to white women. In a study at the University of Arkansas, researchers interviewed 647 female heart attack survivors about their warning symptoms, which often went unheeded as they occurred months or even years before the attack. Black and white women both said that, in looking back, they remembered experiencing fatigue, sleep disturbances, shortness of breath, anxiety, and indigestion prior to their heart attacks. But black women seem to have more headaches, vision problems, and breathing difficulties prior to their heart attacks—and to suffer these symptoms more severely—than do other women.[12]

Doctors are in denial, too. In 1996, a Gallup survey revealed that half the primary care physicians polled thought breast cancer and osteoporosis were greater health threats than heart disease to women over age fifty (they were wrong).

Compounding the situation (and in part explaining it) is a general prejudice—among the lay public and physicians alike—toward interpreting a woman's symptoms as indicative of stress or anxiety rather than disease.[13] A 1999 study cited in *The New England Journal of Medicine* was especially distressing in its demonstration of how doctors sometimes make clinical decisions. While viewing videotapes of actors in a hospital setting, 720 primary care physicians were asked to decide which of the alleged patients should be referred for heart disease testing or treatment (the physicians knew they were watching actors). Patients played by women were recommended for testing 40 percent less frequently than patients played by men, even though they were scripted to complain of identical chest discomfort.[14]

Clearly, female heart patients are not being treated aggressively enough, and many people both inside and outside the medical community are outraged about it. A 1998 study of the records of more than 350,000 patients at more than 1,200 hospitals found that women were less likely to undergo cardiac catheterization, balloon angioplasty, and bypass surgery, and significantly less likely to receive thrombolytic (clot-busting) drugs after a heart attack.[15] And another 1998 study found that exercise stress tests were given nearly twice as often to men as to women.[16] We don't know why women are receiving less aggressive care than men, but we can infer that:

- Many physicians tend to interpret women's symptoms as emotional rather than cardiovascular in nature.
- Too few physicians are aware of the threat that heart illness poses to women.
- Women are not taking their symptoms seriously enough to report them when they should.

But physicians, patients, and even the media are becoming more aware: three weeks after this book was first published in April 2003, *Time* magazine got the word out with a cover story on women and heart disease. And advocacy groups are (wo)manning the barricades against prejudices that keep women from receiving the heart care they need. One of the best is WomenHeart, the National Coalition for Women with Heart Disease, founded by women with heart illness and devoted to providing information on the need for early detection, accurate diagnosis, and proper treatment of the condition (see p. 257). This group and others listed in the Resources section are staffed by energetic activists committed to saving lives—but they can't find you. You have to pick up the phone, get on the Web, or drop them a line. You have to *do* something.

Here's what else you have to do:

- If you're a woman with heart illness, you must be vigilant about attending to your symptoms and insisting on proper medical care and follow-up.
- If you're someone who cares about a woman with heart illness, do become an advocate for her in her quest for competent medical care.
- If you're a woman, *don't deny bodily symptoms—particularly ones that may be related to heart illness.* Even women who are healthy and have no history of cardiovascular problems can develop them. Remember: *all known cardiac risk factors combined account for only 75 percent of the diagnosed cases of heart illness*—the other 25 percent remain of uncertain origin. Heart disease can hit anyone, and we don't know why.
- If you're a man and care about a woman with heart illness, see the above.

STAGE II: CREATING A COPING STRATEGY

Once your condition has stabilized and your fears of imminent death have eased, you start asking what happens next. As you and your family contemplate the answers to these questions—and you should ask lots of them—you will, as a team, start to develop a plan for coping with the illness.

Most families enter this stage within a few days of the onset of the illness, either while the patient is in the hospital or shortly after they receive the diagnosis. Other families don't start developing a coping plan until the patient comes home. While this is a relatively brief phase, it is crucial for both the patient and family.

It is at this point that you begin to understand what heart illness is and what your recovery and treatment will involve. At first, you may be confused and overwhelmed by information. Because your emotions may be fluctuating wildly, you may not be able to focus on what you need to do to

A PATIENT'S RIGHTS

Regardless of your age, sex, race, religion, ethnic heritage, or income, you have the right to:

- Receive considerate, courteous care.
- Be fully informed of your medical condition and the treatment options available to you, and to have this explained in terms you can understand.
- Know the names and qualifications of the people who provide your treatment.
- Help make decisions that affect your treatment.
- Seek second, third, or even fourth opinions, and to change doctors if you are not satisfied with your care.
- Put into place the necessary legal directives to ensure your preferences are honored if you are not able to care for yourself.
- Review your medical records and to request that anything you do not understand be explained to you.
- Receive reasonably prompt responses to your questions and requests.
- Receive reasonable continuity of care. If, for example, your cardiologist retires, he or she should refer your case to another physician who will then care for you.
- Receive full explanations about research studies your doctor may invite you to join, and to continued medical care if you decline to participate. Pharmaceutical companies sometimes ask physicians to recruit patients for drug studies. If your doctor offers you such an opportunity and you don't wish to participate, your declining should have no effect on your relationship with the doctor, nor on the quality of care he or she provides.
- Receive answers to and explanations of questions you may have about fees charged for medical services and reimbursements made by your insurer.
- Have your privacy and confidentiality respected. Your medical records are not your property, but you do have a right to see them, to receive a copy of them, and to have them explained to you. Doctors should release them to others without your written permission *only* if they are required to do so by law (for review by insurers or to address public health concerns). Otherwise, they should *never* be released without your written permission.

get well. For example, a nutritionist may be offering tips on heart-healthy cooking when all you can think about is when you'll be able to return to work and start bringing in money again. Or an exercise therapist might be praising the benefits of a brisk daily walk when you're quietly panicked about whether you'll be able to resume your sex life (yes, you will). When heart disease has shaken your world and you're trying to reorient yourself to the new terrain, it's sometimes hard to grasp information that doesn't pertain to the step you're trying to take. If you find yourself overwhelmed by advice, facts, and statistics, remember that *things will eventually get back to normal*—albeit a new normal—and you will soon pull yourself together.

At this stage, powerful emotions surge to the surface. You and your family begin contemplating how the illness will affect your lives, both as individuals and as a group, and this inevitably opens a vein of grief. Many of my patients report feeling profoundly sad upon learning they have heart disease. This sadness is actually grief for their lost sense of invulnerability. None of us is invulnerable, of course, but heart disease is visceral, in-your-face proof of your mortality, and a humbling loss of innocence.

Grief is intensely personal, and each person handles it differently. Some families are outwardly emotional and experience a wailing-and-gnashing-of-teeth variety of mourning; others report a pervasive melancholy that descends, like a blue mantle, and envelops the entire family. Many patients become obsessed with thoughts about life in general and their lives in particular—past, present, and future. The grieving may even continue into the next stage of your recovery, but you should be aware that now, the second stage, is when it starts.

Even when you understand what has happened to you and what the next steps in your recovery will be, you may not feel confident that you can cope. This insecurity is compounded by the fact that many heart patients are released from the hospital after only a few days, often before they feel ready to return home. With the health insurance situation in our country being what it is, this discharge-'em-quick policy will probably not change anytime soon. So you need to put your energy into adjusting to your new life and focus on two concepts:

1. You have made it this far.
2. You should have some idea of what you will and will not be doing for the next few days, weeks, and months.

You should also know you are an active participant in your recovery and have certain inalienable rights with regard to your medical care. A list of those rights appears on page 16.[17] Read it and reread it until you believe it.

STAGE III: HANDLING THE HOMECOMING BLUES

Reality sets in: you're home, you're on your own, and you're expected to surf a bewildering wave of emotions, anxieties, and procedures. No longer are nurses and doctors checking, monitoring, and calming you, wielding clipboards, stethoscopes, and official, efficient cheer. Now *you* have to decide what you can and cannot do, and you may feel under-qualified for the job. What used to be simple is suddenly unbearably complex; making a bed, a doctor's appointment, or even a tuna-fish sandwich can overwhelm you and bring you to tears. You feel childish and emotional and terribly alone. But you're not: depression is a normal part of recovery, and it comes in many forms. It's all part of creating a new normal for yourself: establishing a new set of attitudes and expectations that redefine what normal means in your life.

HOMECOMING IS HUMBLING

Carlos is the kind of guy you'd like to have around in an emergency, a man who likes to take control of situations and bend them to his will. A forty-six-year-old New Yorker, Carlos had come south as vice-president of human relations for a major restaurant chain. As time passed, I learned he was competitive and driven—especially when it came to driving. He admitted he drove like a lunatic; he would compete with himself to see how quickly he could cover the sixty-mile commute to his office. His record: thirty-nine minutes (about ninety miles per hour). In one of these contests, he veered off the road and his blood pressure spiked high enough to burst blood vessels in his eye.

No one was more surprised than Carlos the day his chest seized up and the paramedics came crashing into his office; two days later, he was scheduled for quadruple coronary artery bypass graft surgery (CABG), popularly known as a quadruple bypass. Carlos was determined to prevail; once the sedation wore off, he started pestering nurses and doctors about when he might go home. He soon got his wish, but homecoming wasn't what he thought it would be:

"Coming home was a setback. My lungs filled with fluid and I couldn't talk for days because the tube they stuck down my throat during surgery had damaged my vocal cords. And I was tired all the time, unbelievably tired. I remember one day my reading lamp burned out and I went to change the bulb. By the time I walked to the garage, found a bulb, got it out of the package, walked back to the den, unscrewed the old bulb and put in the new one, I thought I'd keel over.

"Even worse, I felt isolated recovering in the house. My wife worked it out so she could work from home a few days a week. But after three days of that, I sent her back to the office. I didn't want her around all day, seeing me so weak and out of control.

FEMALE HEART PATIENTS ARE SELDOM HOMECOMING QUEENS, EVEN THOUGH THEY NEED TO BE

Women's homecoming experiences differ from men's in a very important way: they get less support. Husbands of heart attack patients provide less hands-on help and participate less in recovery than wives do.[18] Plus, more female than male patients face recovery on their own because women tend to outlive their spouses more than men do. Women are more likely than men to insist that their families not be inconvenienced for the sake of their rehabilitation, resulting in family dynamics that are less oriented toward the patient's needs than they should be.

A woman with heart illness often finds herself marinating in a potent brew of shock, anger, loneliness, and stress:

- **Shock** because our culture still downplays the epidemic of heart illness among women.

- **Anger** because, after years of pleading with the people she loves to take care of themselves, *she's* the one who got sick.

- **Loneliness** because her family is less likely to provide the support and care she needs.

- **Stress** because her domestic responsibilities don't come with a disability plan. Many women—even those with demanding careers—are the organizational and spiritual hubs of their families. When they're out of commission, everyone else can be thrown into utter disarray, compounding the patient's anguish.

"Things got better slowly—very slowly. Once my lungs cleared and I could breathe better, I started walking every day. That was good—I burned off some energy and ran into a few neighbors I hadn't seen in a while. But what I was thinking about most was getting back to work—and I did, just as soon as I could."

Homecoming blues usually descend during a patient's first few weeks at home after a hospital stay. An Australian study followed thirty-eight heart attack survivors for three weeks after they returned home. Almost all of them experienced periods of anxiety and depression because they were uncertain about the progress of their recovery and worried about suffering another heart attack or serious health problem.[19] And researchers have begun paying special attention to bypass patients, who seem particularly vulnerable to severe bouts of depression after surgery. While we don't yet have definitive statistics, we do know that between 30 and 75 percent or more of bypass patients struggle with intense melancholy after the operation. And, while most depressed bypass patients do recover emotionally within six months of the surgery, they say those early weeks of paralyzing gloom are profoundly painful to endure.[20]

Homecoming is a challenging experience for families, too. Surveys consistently show that a heart patient's loved ones find the first days of homecoming to be a difficult and frightening time, and that only one out of five caregivers feels ready to welcome the patient home and properly care for him or her.[21] If you're like most patients, when you returned home you and your family probably craved more information than you received about heart illness in general, your condition specifically, and what sort of rehabilitation plan you would need. People want to know how long it will take to recover, what side effects the medications may have, how the family can help the patient cope, and what patients should do—as well as what they should not do—during the first month of recovery.

A hazard of this early adjustment time is the urge of family members to do too much for the patient, or, in the case of Rena and Tom, to prevent the patient from doing things she or he is fully capable of. When Rena's grown children banded together and defeated her valiant attempt at spring cleaning—her first deliberate effort to conduct a new normal activity—they thought they were protecting their mother. Instead, they denied her the opportunity to feel capable and useful—feelings that can be in short supply for a new heart patient.

As you may have already learned, the first month at home is a time of trial and error—lots of error. Because you haven't yet learned what you can and cannot safely do, you're probably constantly asking yourself, "Am I doing all right?" In the meantime, the person or people you live with are probably lurking in the shadows, monitoring your every move: "Do you think it's okay for you to do that? Have you taken your medicine? How are you feeling? Why don't you let me do that for you?" These reminders and offers of help may at first soothe and reassure you, but it's almost certain that they'll soon become irritating and you'll find yourself growing testy with the people who are trying to help. The best way to handle this is to let overeager helpers know how their efforts are affecting you tactfully, rather than lash out and bite the hands that feed you, drive you, and bring you your medicine. (I have devoted Chapter 4 to ways to handle this kind of situation, as well as others.)

Early homecoming is also a time when the needs of patients and family members tend to diverge. During the crisis stage, when you're in the hospital and your family gathers around, everyone's energy is focused on you—whether you'll survive, what the illness means, what treatment you'll require, and how to get you well again. But once the crisis passes and you come home, the personal needs of family members—especially those of the primary caregiver—begin to surface. As you've probably learned, family tensions will develop if these needs aren't acknowledged and addressed.

Here are five factors that commonly complicate homecoming blues, and hints for handling them:

1. Unfamiliar physical and emotional symptoms
2. Temporary or ongoing cognitive difficulties
3. Coping overkill
4. Grief
5. Posttraumatic stress disorder (PTSD)

Let's go over these one by one.

UNFAMILIAR PHYSICAL AND EMOTIONAL SYMPTOMS

In the early stages of recovery, you may experience unfamiliar sensations. You may feel a strange combination of fear, weakness, fatigue, and helplessness. It might take you all day to complete household chores you used to zip through before lunch. If you find yourself moving very slowly or going through periods of depression, weeping, social withdrawal, or obsessive anxiety about dying, remember that these are normal during the early stages of heart disease—painful, yes; frightening, yes; dangerous, *no*.

As I mentioned earlier, if you've had bypass surgery, you'll face unique homecoming challenges. First, you're likely to be surprised at how long it takes to recover from the effects of the surgery, which could include the following:

- Feeling as if your heart is loose in your chest
- Shoulder and back strain
- Numbness in the chest
- Pain if leg or sternum incisions are rubbed
- Chest discomfort, especially when the humidity drops
- Sleeplessness
- Anxiety
- Depression
- Dizziness
- Inability to concentrate
- Poor memory, particularly about events during your hospital stay
- Loss of taste for food, which may be due to the effects of medication or trauma to taste buds from the respirator mouthpiece (this condition is usually temporary)

Many bypass patients experience a condition called **postpump syndrome.** This refers to memory and concentration problems that may be related to a combination of medication, stress, and hardening of the arteries—all of which may affect brain functioning. There is also evidence that tiny air bubbles may pass through filters in the heart-lung machine during surgery, and these bubbles may temporarily interfere with the supply of oxygen to the brain.

An alternate explanation implicates the clamps used during surgery to block blood flow from the aorta. When the surgery is over and the clamps are removed, fragments of plaque—fibrous tissue that causes hardening of the arteries—may break loose and block portions of blood vessels, disrupting blood flow to the brain.[22]

Here's the great news: these memory and concentration problems typically begin to subside within six months of surgery and are usually gone within a year. In a 1996 study, researchers evaluated 2,108 bypass patients at twenty-four hospitals, and found that only 3 percent of them suffered symptoms of serious brain complications such as paralysis caused by stroke or milder complications such as confusion or memory loss.[23] So if you're having these symptoms, chances are excellent that you won't have them much longer; they usually subside after the first few months. You can hasten their departure by attending rehabilitation classes; likewise, the more unhealthy behaviors you indulge in, such as smoking, overeating, and loafing all day in the La-Z-Boy, the more likely these symptoms are to linger. Moreover, many patients who report symptoms after six months are likely suffering more from effects of depression than a brain syndrome. A study in *The Journal of Thoracic Cardiovascular Surgery* reported that approximately four out of ten bypass patients were found to have been depressed *before* their surgery, indicating that their postsurgical cognitive difficulties may not have been due to the surgery at all but rather to a very treatable condition: depression.[24]

TEMPORARY OR ONGOING COGNITIVE DIFFICULTIES

The brain requires a constant flow of oxygenated blood to function properly. Many factors that cause heart disease, as well as some of its treatments, can impede this flow, resulting in anoxia, an absence of blood in the brain, or hypoxia, reduced oxygen supply to the brain. If your brain receives less oxygen than it needs, you may experience cognitive deficits that prevent you from thinking as clearly as you used to. As you just read, bypass patients commonly go through this as a result of the surgery.

While these cognitive problems are not unique to the homecoming period, this is usually when they are first identified and most intensely experienced. Whether you're the patient or a family member, it's a good idea for you to know what to expect, so here is a brief summary of the cognitive problems that most often afflict heart patients, the conditions with which the problems are associated, and how various treatments for heart illness affect the brain. While many of these deficits are temporary and relatively minor in medical terms, their effects on   your ability to cope with daily life may seem major to you. If, for example, you've always had a crackerjack memory and suddenly have trouble recalling people's names, the havoc this wreaks on your self-image will probably dwarf the physiological short-circuit that caused it. The point is, even if your doctor warns that you may experience "small" alterations in the way your mind works, they may not seem so little to you—or to your family—and will take some getting used to.

Here are some of the most common cognitive deficits and their symptoms: [25]

- **Attention problems.** You have these if you have difficulty with the following activities:
  - Paying attention for extended periods of time
  - Paying attention to some things while screening out others
  - Tracking several things at once, such as boiling a pot of potatoes while watching the playoffs on TV and remembering to take your medication (also known as mental flexibility)
  - Completing complex tasks that require you to simultaneously pay attention, scan, shift focus, and perform motor skills (driving, for example)
- **Memory problems.** May affect either short- or long-term memory.
- **Perceptual problems.** A decline in the skills that help you perceive your surroundings, such as the ability to identify a person or thing by looking at it.
- **Abstract reasoning problems.** A decline in the ability to solve problems by integrating new information with old or grasping complex concepts.

Here are some common heart conditions and the cognitive problems associated with them:

- **High blood pressure.** If you have hypertension and don't treat it, you may have problems with memory, abstract reasoning, attention, and learning.
- **Elevated cholesterol level.** This in itself does not affect the way your mind works but does increase your risk of developing hardening of the arteries, whose sufferers manifest cognitive deficits from middle age on.
- **Myocardial infarction, or heart attack.** Between 30 and 40 percent of heart attack survivors have problems with memory, disorientation, and fine motor skills in the months after the event. Others have problems with manual dexterity, verbal communication, recall of newly acquired information, and mental flexibility. Serious cognitive impairment, or dementia, is particularly common in elderly women who have suffered more than one heart attack.
- **Sudden cardiac arrest (SCA).** People who suffer this syndrome commonly experience cognitive difficulties, especially long-term memory loss. They also endure diminished ability to recognize familiar objects and sometimes begin to exhibit traits associated with relationship distress, including apathy, irritability, and limited insight and empathy. (For more on SCA, see Chapter 12.)

CHECK YOUR BLOOD PRESSURE!

If you haven't had your blood pressure checked in the last year, do it now: your levels may be higher than they should be. In May 2003, the National Heart, Lung, and Blood Institute (NHLBI) released new guidelines for diagnosing hypertension, and what used to be considered acceptable is no longer good enough. In the past, a blood pressure level of 120 systolic/80 diastolic was called normal; now it's called prehypertension, because research shows that people who fall into this new category are at increased risk of developing hypertension. According to NHLBI, patients whose blood pressure levels are in the 130–139/80–89 range are twice as likely to develop hypertension as those whose levels are lower.[26] And even if your levels are normal—according to the new guidelines, up to 119/79—you should still exercise, keep your weight down, watch how much salt and alcohol you ingest, and manage stress, anger, and depression. New data show that people who have normal blood pressure levels at age fifty-five still have a 90 percent lifetime risk of developing hypertension.[27]

- **Heart failure.** Chronic heart failure leads to an ongoing oxygen drought in the brain, which in turn provokes a wide range of cognitive impairments. (See Chapter 11.)
- **Arrhythmia.** Patients with a long history of arrhythmia are more likely to suffer from stroke and ongoing diminished blood supply to the brain than those with normal heart rhythms. Over years, this can result in dementia. Early detection and treatment, especially with a pacemaker, may halt the deterioration (see p. 26).

Finally, here are some notes on how common treatments for heart disease affect the brain:

- **Vasodilating medications.** Drugs (and other treatments) that expand blood vessels increase the flow of oxygenated blood to the brain. It follows that they might also improve cognitive functioning, and this is often the case.
- **Antihypertensive medications.** Drugs to treat high blood pressure, especially beta-blockers, seem to improve long-term memory in some patients. They seem to have no negative effects on brain functioning.

- **CABG (bypass surgery).** The risk of neuropsychological problems associated with bypass surgery rises along with the patient's age, the severity of the disease, and the number of vessels that must be bypassed during the surgery.

- **Pacemaker.** A study of 450 patients who received pacemakers to correct arrhythmias showed that more than 60 percent of them experienced at least a partial reversal of their cognitive deficits—very good news indeed.[28]

- **Carotid endarterectomy (surgical procedure to remove atherosclerotic plaque from the walls of the carotid artery).** The purpose of this procedure is to rid a patient's artery of plaque before enough accumulates to clog it and cause a stroke. Ironically, it has long been worrisome to doctors, who have feared that loosened plaque might be swept away to the brain, where it could cause greater damage. But research indicates otherwise: the cognitive abilities of people who have had the procedure don't seem to change either way.

COPING OVERKILL

When you or someone you love is diagnosed with heart disease, a swarm of fears can descend upon the household. People tend to call up their most deeply ingrained coping habits when they're afraid. This sometimes causes a syndrome I call coping overkill, in which the patient, family members, or both turn into the heart-health police. Believing they must now be paragons of healthy living, they become preoccupied with catching themselves and others making mistakes. (This is as unnecessary as it is unwise, and I'll discuss it later.)

The coping overkill syndrome has many varieties, which tend to resemble exaggerated versions of the personalities involved. A moody woman who's suffering from coping overkill might bristle at a simple request. A man who is suspicious by nature might question the intentions of his physicians and loved ones. In some cases, the primary caretaker focuses almost exclusively on others, denying his or her own needs to the point of exhaustion. I've also seen this happen to the family peacemaker, often a grown daughter or son who acts as a go-between for emotionally volatile family members.

Any coping pattern that becomes obsessive will exhaust you and increase family tensions. If someone close to you has veered into coping overkill, ask him or her to sit down with you and discuss the situation. If you're the one who's suffering from the syndrome, first admit it to yourself, then admit it to the patient or the other family members, and then, finally, figure out what personal needs you've been ignoring and set about attending to them.

Grief

When you're diagnosed with a chronic illness, the future looks a lot different than it did the day before (and usually not as good). In the early weeks after diagnosis, it is common for heart patients and the people who love them to feel and act as though someone has died. If this has happened to you, you know how hard it can be to distinguish homecoming blues from this paralyzing, all-encompassing grief.

Here are some manifestations of the grief that often accompanies homecoming:

- **Denial:** "They're making a big deal out of nothing. I'm sure it was my stomach, not my heart."
- **Anger:** "Would you just leave me alone? I don't want to talk about this right now."
- **Sadness:** "I'm feeling much too depressed to leave the house. Maybe I'll go out with you tomorrow."
- **Confusion:** "I can't keep track of all this information. I don't even know what pills I'm taking or when I'm supposed to take them—it's too much for me."
- **Despair:** "Oh, Lord! I can't handle this . . . everything's different . . . I don't know what to do."
- **Guilt:** "If only I'd quit smoking when you told me to. Now I've ruined both our lives."
- **Bargaining:** "If I live a perfectly healthy life and do everything I'm supposed to, maybe this will all go away."

If any of this sounds familiar, take heart: grief is temporary (I know it doesn't feel that way, but that's the nature of grief). With support and time, it lifts. Make sure you have someone to remind you that these devastating feelings will indeed pass and that you're on this journey for the long haul. The key is to express your feelings, not hold them in.

Posttraumatic Stress Disorder (PTSD)

You may read this material about depression and think, "Hey—that's not me. The hospital was a breeze; I'm still my usual cheery self!" Please take a break from your victory dance long enough to read this section, because you may not be in the clear just yet (on the other hand, if you are, terrific!—but read this section anyway). Research shows that as many as 20 percent of heart attack patients who seem unfazed by the hospital experience develop emotional problems about four months after it ends.[27] One explanation for this alarming statistic is that many patients experience undiagnosed (and untreated) posttraumatic stress disorder when they come home from the hospital.

Here is how it happens. Many patients become severely disoriented and confused in the alien environment of the hospital or from physical trauma of surgery and recovery. This often occurs while they are in the Intensive Care Unit (ICU) or the Coronary Care Unit (CCU). You may have experienced this disorientation if you had any of the following symptoms:

- Confusion about objective reality (what day it is, what preceded your arrival in the ICU or CCU, and so on)
- Trouble thinking in a logical way
- Seeing or hearing things that are either unreal or not present, or having hallucinations
- Fearing that medical personnel or others are or were trying to harm you
- Memory lapses
- Lack of trust or suspiciousness
- Irritability
- Rapid mood changes

Medication may add to the confusion. During this initial stage of recovery, patients are often dosed with sedatives that may cloud their judgment and memory. They may also receive pain medication after surgery that limits their tolerance for light and noise and clouds their ability to think clearly.

In the past, about one third of recovering patients experienced such confusion; with patients over the age of sixty, the fraction was higher. Happily, these figures have improved markedly in recent years, probably because we now move heart surgery patients out of intensive care more swiftly than we used to.

While the confusion can be painful for both patient and loved ones, the good news is it usually doesn't last long and seems to depart on its own. But it can leave emotional scars: if you've experienced postoperative disorientation, you may be left with partial memories of the scary time, confusion about why it happened, and fear that it may happen again. This is where posttraumatic stress disorder creeps in—when you have frightening flashbacks about what you've been through well after you've been through it. You can recognize the disorder by a combination of some or all of the following symptoms:

- Upsetting memories of the cardiac event that keep popping into your mind
- Disturbing dreams about the event
- Obsessive thoughts about upsetting details of the event
- A tendency to weep or cry
- Anxiety
- Sleep problems
- Acting or feeling as if the event were happening again or just about to happen again
- Having a startle response—for example, jumping when the phone rings or when you hear a siren
- Avoidance behaviors—for instance, driving four miles out of your way to avoid passing the hospital
- Difficulty controlling your mood or an inability to concentrate

If you've experienced one or more of these symptoms, it's possible that you're suffering from posttraumatic stress disorder, or PTSD. And if you're close to someone who has PTSD, you know that, without meaning to, family members may sometimes complicate the problem.

When a heart patient has PTSD, his or her mate, children, and other loved ones are accosted by an upsetting view of the person they love: the patient is confused, doesn't make sense, is not acting like him- or herself, and may even lash out in anger and despair. Not knowing what to say or do, family members often shy away from talking with the patient about what actually happened in the hospital, figuring that things will work out on their own if they avoid the obvious issue: the trauma of the cardiac event and what came after.

Avoiding the issue is usually a mistake. Patients recover faster and more completely in an atmosphere of openness and acceptance, when they are encouraged to talk about their feelings with people who love and support them. Evasive comments such as "Things did get sort of out of hand those first few days" will probably leave the patient silently worrying about what actually happened that he or she can't remember. And silence is equally bad if not worse, as it exaggerates the patient's feeling of isolation and inhibits his or her ability to acknowledge, understand, and cope with the disorder.

If you think you are suffering from PTSD, here are seven steps you can take right now to help you get the problem under control:

1. **Acknowledge that something very frightening happened.** Losing your ability to think straight or take care of yourself—even temporarily—is upsetting.

2. **Know that you are not alone.** About one third of heart patients go through this.

3. Be reassured that **these reactions have nothing whatsoever to do with your overall mental health.** The symptoms you are experiencing are temporary stress reactions to the extraordinary situation you faced in the hospital. Traumatic experiences often affect the mind the way a power surge affects a computer: they can shock the operating system—your brain—into temporary blowout mode, short-circuiting its electrical connections and disabling you from thinking the way you typically do (makes you wish you could attach a surge protector to your head, doesn't it?).

4. Remember that **for the vast majority of people, this is a temporary condition, and, once it's over, it does not recur.**

5. That said, remember also that **it is normal to have flashbacks (psychological relivings of the event) or bouts of emotion after surgery** that might not make sense to you. This is because you may have partial memories of what you heard, thought, or saw as you were drifting in and out of awareness during and after surgery.

6. **Don't hold it all inside—talk about what you experienced.** The more you talk about these confusing episodes, the more love and support you'll get from the people around you, and the sooner you'll recover.

7. **If you don't feel significantly better within four to six weeks, talk with your doctor.** You may need professional counseling.

All too often, patients at risk of developing adjustment problems slip through the many cracks in our country's health care system. We know from research that certain heart patients are highly likely to struggle upon returning home and to have a poorer quality of life six months to a year later. Especially at risk are people who show high levels of anxiety and depression in the hospital, those who are suffering from angina (chest discomfort or pain) when they are discharged, those who are younger than sixty-five, and those who lack a support system of either family, friends, or a combination of both. This last group consists mostly of patients who live alone and don't have a life partner or close friend with whom they share an intimate emotional bond and to whom they can turn for comfort and support. If any of these descriptions sounds like you, **please, get counseling. Tell a physician, nurse, pastor, or someone else that you've been diagnosed with heart disease and need support. Doing this can determine not only how happy you are, but whether or not you survive.**[30]

STAGE IV: LEARNING TO LIVE WITH HEART DISEASE

You don't have to struggle against heart illness; you can live with it. Many people even thrive with it. Most take between six and twelve months to get somewhat comfortable with their new, heart-healthy way of life (not totally comfortable, but on the way to comfortable).

Give yourself a chance to get comfortable with living in a heart-healthy way; it's a big transition to your new normal. Remember that a large part of the transition is learning to talk to the people you love and live with about what you're going through, what you feel for one another, and what life is *really* about.

BECOME AN INFORMATION MAGNET

Another part of the transition is learning everything you can about living with heart disease. One of the most effective ways to do this is to join a cardiac rehabilitation program, which acquaints people with the psychological and physical ramifications of the illness. An outstanding benefit of cardiac rehabilitation is that it helps you develop a realistic, appropriate recovery plan and teaches you how to measure your success.

And it works! Research shows that people who begin cardiac rehab while they're still in the hospital and continue with the program after they're home—even if it's only for a few months—suffer less anxiety, depression, and disability than those who try to manage on their own. Further, both rehab participants and their families have a fuller understanding of the illness and so are better able as a group to weather the storms that inevitably blow in.[31]

"I HAVEN'T BEEN REFERRED TO REHAB, SO I PROBABLY DON'T NEED IT, RIGHT?"

Wrong! If you haven't been referred to a cardiac rehabilitation program, *find out why.* It may be that your physician has overlooked you as a rehab candidate.

It is alarming but true: two large categories of heart patients tend to be neglected when it comes to rehab referrals: women and the elderly. Recent research shows that physicians are more likely to refer men than women to rehab[32] and to favor younger, healthier patients in general.[33] This happens even though both female patients of all ages and older patients of both sexes have been shown to benefit from cardiac rehab programs every bit as much as do their younger male counterparts.[34]

Here's a glimpse of what researchers have found when they put older heart patients on structured exercise programs:

- **Up to 40 percent improvement in endurance** for women aged sixty-two to eighty-two with coronary heart disease (CHD),[35] with those who were sedentary benefiting the most[36]

- **Improved HDL and LDL levels** (high-density lipoprotein, or "good cholesterol," and low-density lipoprotein, or "bad cholesterol," respectively) over a five-year period for older patients, male and female alike[37]

- **Reduced blood pressure**[38] within eight weeks of starting aerobic activity without increasing aerobic capacity, reducing weight, or changing diet[39]

- **Vast increases in tolerance for exercise** among men and women of every age group, including those over seventy-five, and particularly among those who were in the poorest physical condition when they joined the program[40]

There are more statistics where these came from, but I think you get the point: rehab works, and not just for younger folks in decent shape. **Studies consistently show that the patients with the lowest exercise capacity at the start of a program benefit most from it.**

Participating in a cardiac rehab program is one of the best things you can do to hasten your recovery, and I urge you to do so if you're able. To locate one in your area, get in touch with the American Association of Cardiovascular and Pulmonary Rehabilitation (see Resources for contact information).

FIRST GOALS

One of the first things I teach my patients—and you can count yourself among them—is the importance of organizing their cardiac journeys by setting reachable recovery goals. The best goals are both specific and realistic, because they establish clearly what you must accomplish while ensuring that you have the ability to do it. It's also a good idea to put your goals in writing, as it formalizes your commitment to accomplishing them. And be reassured: You don't have to become a seaweed-eating jogging fanatic to heal your heart. Moderate exercise and reasonable dietary adjustments can provide quantum leaps toward heart health.[41]

We'll focus more on goal-setting later; for now, remember that during the early stages of adjustment, thinking in terms of setting and attaining a goal enables you to chart your progress and develop confidence that living a full life with heart illness is completely possible.

Another habit of well-adjusted heart patients is to note the progress they have made, however small, and reward themselves for it. Reassure yourself that you're doing well by becoming more conscious of your behaviors and acknowledging your healthy ones. You can start by getting into the habit of asking yourself these questions:

1. Did I eat more healthfully today than I typically did before I had heart disease? If not, how can I do better tomorrow?
2. Have I exercised as I planned to this week? If not, what would help me do better next week?
3. Am I developing effective coping behaviors?
4. Am I letting my loved ones know how much they mean to me?

Another characteristic of thriving heart patients is their tendency to think things through when it comes to their heart health. Let's say you live in Chicago, had a heart attack last year, and are planning a trip to Denver to visit your grandchildren. You'd be wise to remember that while you're in Denver, you'll be living a full mile higher than you're accustomed to. This doesn't mean you shouldn't go. It does mean you should be aware that there's less oxygen up there and if your heart starts to pound and you become light-headed, it could be altitude sickness—which you can cure with a couple of whiffs from an oxygen tank—and not another heart attack.[42] (On the other hand, if the grandkids want you to join them on a jaunt up Pikes Peak [altitude 14,110 feet], you should probably develop a previous engagement.)

This is a stage when you and your family should be focusing on treating one another with renewed respect and compassion. When heart disease shocks people into realizing that life is fragile and can be profoundly changed or even snatched away without warning, their behaviors sometimes change: a quiet son may summon the courage to talk about what he's thinking, a controlling matriarch may weep at her feelings of helplessness, an optimistic daughter may turn suddenly cynical, and the curmudgeon of the family may show signs of forgiveness. A person you thought you knew may turn away from you in despair or toward you in desperation. You may feel you don't even know yourself. This too is normal.

When I said it takes about six to twelve months to start adjusting to a heart-healthy way of life, I did not mean that you'll be completely adjusted one calendar year after the cardiac event. As heart illness lasts a lifetime, so does its adjustment period, for both patient and loved ones. And everyone suffers setbacks. What works wonderfully during the early phase of rehabilitation may prove useless later on. Individual difficulties and fresh family dynamics may develop that prompt you to wonder why you never went to live on that desert island you read about in *National Geographic*. This too is normal, although not easy. Because heart disease is with you for life and life means change, you'll need to revise your coping plan as new concerns and issues arise.

COPING TIPS

No matter what stage you've reached in your journey, you're still bound to come up against some obstacles that seem too huge to handle. Here are ten tips to help you cope:

1. **Accept that living well with heart illness requires that you manage your mind, your body, your spirit, and your relationships.** Together, these areas function like a four-legged stool: four strong legs will make you stable, but weakness in any one of them will adversely affect your full recovery. To thrive with heart illness, strive for strength in each of these areas.

2. **Accept that you will need different kinds of support at different stages of your journey.** During a crisis, you will need emotional support that comes from soothing, encouraging words, the loving presence of others, and introspection or prayer. As your recovery progresses, you will need information to help you understand what is happening and how you might cope. And throughout your recovery, you will occasionally need help to accomplish what you used to be able to do on your own, such as getting to the doctor, taking down the drapes, or cleaning out the rain gutters. It's no disgrace to need help. Ask for it when you need it.

3. **Expect setbacks and trust that they will pass.** Understand and accept that living with a chronic illness causes physical and emotional ups and downs. When the ride gets bumpy, hang on and remember that the road will eventually level out.

4. **Don't be afraid of your emotions.** Experiencing painful and powerful emotions is part of coping with illness. While these emotions may hurt, they seldom cause damage. In fact, recent research indicates that heart patients who face and work through painful episodes adjust better to the illness than those who evade their feelings.[43]

5. **Take your medicine!** Making sure you take your medications not only helps you manage the disease; it could save your life. If you have high blood pressure and you take your medicines as prescribed all the time, you're *half as likely* to have a heart attack as someone who takes the medicines only 80 to 90 percent of the time.[44] And if you take your beta-blocker medication just as your doctor told you to, you're also cutting your risk of death by 50 percent.[45]

   With statistics like these, why don't people take their medication? Sometimes it's because they dislike the side effects; often it's because the medication is too costly. If the only thing standing between you and your medication is the cost, please—tell your doctor! This is no time for pride or embarrassment; millions of Americans are unable to afford the prescriptions they need. Your doctor may be able to switch to a less expensive medication or prescribe a generic formula of the more costly name brand. Or you might be eligible for low-cost or even free medications—but you'll never know if you don't ask.

6. **Learn to express yourself.** Being able to talk about your feelings with your family, friends, doctors, and other members of your health care team is a very important part of living well with heart illness. Stifling your feelings—even if you think it will protect your loved ones from seeing you upset and getting upset themselves—will make matters worse, both for you and for them. (For tips on how to express yourself effectively, see Chapter 4.)

7. **Know yourself, and pace your recovery accordingly.** If you want to adjust to this illness, you should start by accepting that you do not have to be perfect. Trying to be the perfect patient or the perfect mate (or daughter, or son, or parent) will make you anxious, irritable, and deplete your strength, as well as place stress on your family. Remember, you're not a contestant on *Beat the Clock*. Take your time. Everyone changes at his or her own pace and in his or her own way. Discover your way and match your pace to it.

8. **Be honest: look inward often, even if you flinch at what you see.** In addition to getting regular checkups from your physician, you must check yourself, also regularly, to see how you're caring for the four areas I mentioned in Coping Tip 1: your mind, your body, your spirit, and your relationships. Accepting that you must manage these areas is one step; maintaining effective management is the next step.

9. **Celebrate your successes.** Well-adjusted heart patients catch themselves doing things right and reward themselves for their efforts. It's easy to dismiss your successes as mere shadows of your previous accomplishments and focus instead on how you're coming up short. Don't fall into this pattern. Every step forward, however small, is a step toward recovery, and a success worth celebrating. You don't have to buy champagne, but you should acknowledge your achievement, if only to yourself.

10. **Draw strength from knowing that you *do* know how to cope with hard times.** It's probably safe to say that you've gone through some tough times. Maybe you've endured a major financial setback, watched a loved one battle a serious illness, or dealt with the death of someone close to you. The point is, you've had some on-the-job training. Give yourself credit for what you've already been through, and use what it taught you to forge ahead.

That's the image I want you to burn into your mind: forging ahead, one foot in front of the other, sometimes steadily, sometimes not so steadily, but moving, always moving forward in your journey of recovery. You *can* make it—and you will—if you keep your head up, your eyes open, and your hands clasped firmly with those of the people you care about. You're all in this together, as you'll see in Chapter 3.

Chapter Three

YOU CAN'T DO IT ALONE

(Heart Illness Is No Place for Hermits)

Some days, my wife, Mary, and I have the best jobs in the world. As partners in our counseling practice, we spend many hours meeting with heart patients and the people who love them and live with them. On the best days, we leave work better people than when we arrived, ennobled by listening to our clients talk about how they help one another navigate the unknown waters of cardiac recovery. We hear stories of women stopping short in the bedroom doorway, silently watching their husbands weep for the first time in forty years and tactfully determining whether they need privacy or comfort. We hear about men up at one in the morning ironing the Thanksgiving tablecloth, protecting their wives from the pressure they'd feel to get everything done before the kids arrive, pumpkin pie in hand, the next day.

We watch our clients fumble for tissues as they tell us how they are learning to listen, really listen, when the person they love needs to talk about the illness that has rocked their lives. We nod as we hear about children who allow their parents to let some menial tasks slide and still know the home is intact: a high school junior who skips the movies with his buddies to shop for groceries at night; a thirteen-year-old who volunteers to do the whole family's laundry instead of just her own, and her six-year-old brother who does his best to match the socks when they come out of the dryer.

We are moved by these stories of ordinary people in extraordinary circumstances, people we like to think of as household heroes. In our world, heroes are people who create safe spaces for others, gifts of protection where a person can feel safe while navigating his or her recovery. When someone creates a safe space for a person with heart disease, both are bound by an elastic, caring connection that helps them bounce back, reclaim hope, and continue to find meaning in life, even when they face a barrage of stresses.

But we have also seen many families flounder in anger and confusion in the wake of heart disease. We have listened to intelligent, educated men and women who refuse to see any hope in their situation or to grasp the lifelines we toss them. We have seen grown children refuse to acknowledge the seriousness of their parents' illness and deny them the support they need. We have watched couples—married and unmarried, older and younger, straight and gay—bicker over issues worthy of a couple of four-year-olds because they cannot get beyond their rage and resentment that this has happened to them.

Some relationships and families weather the hurricane of heart illness; others blow apart. People blame themselves, then turn on the people around them. A man accuses his wife of not caring enough to remind him to take his medication; then, when she calls out that it's time for his pills, he complains that she's nagging. Two women in a twenty-year relationship find themselves worrying and arguing for the first time about money, their careers, and the future. Just when they need each other's love and support the most, they devolve into a spiral of stress, struggle, and isolation. Or, in an ironic twist, family members try so hard to shield the heart patient from everyday worries, they make the patient worry even more.

"DON'T TELL DAD—HE MIGHT WORRY"

The first time I saw Maria Hinson, she reminded me of a small, wary bird. She rose from a chair in my waiting room and met my gaze with a weak smile; her eyes, though intense, were set within dark, bluish circles. She looked about sixty-five, although I knew she was a dozen years younger. Her family doctor had referred her to me for help with stress and exhaustion: for more than nine months, she had been crippled by a combination of migraine headaches and insomnia. As she walked into my office, I noticed the prominent bones of her wrists and ankles, angular evidence of the weight she had lost. It was clear to me that Maria was depressed. Yet she was supposed to be the healthy one—her husband was the heart patient, not she.

As we began, Maria said she enjoyed life, was happily married to a loving husband, and the proud mother of a college-age son. After a while she admitted that three years earlier she'd been very scared when her husband, Henry, had suffered a moderately serious heart attack. She emphasized that Henry's recovery had been uncomplicated—so much so, in fact, that he had breezed through triple coronary artery bypass surgery not long after the heart attack. When I commented that heart disease can be tough on families, Maria smiled tightly and said that she and her family had made it through just fine.

As we talked, I slowly realized that Maria did not see the connection between Henry's heart illness and her own struggles. Whenever her husband's name came up, she assured me that he was making excellent progress. She mentioned several times that she and her son had adjusted their lives and the family's activities to accommodate Henry's illness.

I prodded further and asked what adjustments they had made. Maria said that Henry had wrestled with depression before the heart attack and admitted that even after twenty-six years of marriage, he was still a bit of a mystery to her. On the one hand, he was a dynamo, an ambitious, self-made man. He had built a successful heating and air-conditioning business, house by house and vent by vent, and Maria spoke of his pride in the family's prosperity.

But Henry was also a chronic worrier, prone to periods of depression in which he would quietly obsess about anything and everything that might go wrong. Maria said Henry had been particularly concerned when their son, John, had decided to switch his major from business to psychology. From the time John had been five years old, Henry had taken him on weekend work calls, teaching him about ducts and compressors, envisioning the day he would turn the business over to his son, their only child. Now Henry wasn't sure that would happen and worried that the business would collapse when he retired. At this point Maria drew herself up, took a deep breath, and gazed directly into my eyes as she spoke.

"My son and I took charge of the situation and came up with our own preventive medicine strategy: to protect Henry from stress—*all* stress."

I listened as Maria described her strategy. John, who had been a junior in college at the time of his father's heart attack, had withdrawn from school and come home to help his mother run the business. Between them, they took calls from customers, ordered equipment, and supervised Henry's workmen as best they could.

In addition, Maria acted as a buffer between Henry and the world beyond the den, where he sat in his favorite chair most of the time, reading the newspaper or watching television. Every morning she waited for the mail to arrive, intercepted the bills, and stashed them in a kitchen cabinet. If Henry dozed off for twenty minutes, she'd run to the kitchen, write out a few checks, and have them stamped and in her purse before he woke up. Maria was especially proud of what she had done when the furnace burned out: she and John had spoken to Henry's workmen, ordered a new furnace,

THRIVING WITH HEART DISEASE

.and arranged for them to install it, "without bothering Henry with the details."

Meanwhile, Maria made sure she did not alarm Henry with any mention of her headaches, insomnia, or weight loss. Once, when Henry remarked that she was looking a little gaunt, Maria told him how pleased she was that he'd noticed her diet was working.

I asked Maria how this antistress strategy was working. All at once her eyes grew wet. Maria whispered that she was growing more and more concerned about her husband. Henry seemed miserable. He had aged since the heart attack and surgery; he wasn't yet sixty, but his hair was completely gray now, and he shuffled his feet when he walked. He seemed uninterested in life; not exactly depressed, but melancholy and unresponsive. He seldom laughed and was withdrawing from the family more and more. Maria told me she ached for the romance and intimacy she and Henry used to enjoy. At the end of the session, Maria agreed that I should meet with Henry next.

A week later, I greeted Henry Hinson in my waiting room. A tall, solid man, he wore a navy blue blazer and gray slacks and had a powerful presence but at the same time seemed unsure of himself. He couldn't quite look me in the eye when we shook hands and hesitated slightly when I invited him into my office. His combination of poise and awkwardness reminded me of how a football coach acts when his team has lost a big game.

Henry did not like the spectator role his wife and son had assigned him and spoke with more than a touch of annoyance:

> *"Yes, I had a heart attack and bypass surgery three years ago, but my wife and son act as if I'd died three years ago. Bills come to the house, and Maria hides them somewhere in the kitchen. My son, who didn't know a profit-and-loss statement from a lost-and-found station, all of a sudden quit college and moved into my office at the building that I built for the business that I created—and he didn't even talk to me about it first.*
>
> *"And here's the kicker. The furnace burned out four months ago. Does anybody tell me? That's my business, right? I know heating, I know my house—I know what to do better than anyone. So you think they'd sit down and ask my opinion. But do they? No! They go behind my back, to my own men, and ask them what to do. They made the right decision; they bought the right furnace and installed it just fine. But I can't tell you how bad that made me feel—how useless, how ridiculous.*
>
> *"Now, don't get me wrong: I love my wife and my son, and I appreciate what they're trying to do for me. But I keep thinking they must know something about my condition that I don't know—that I must be a lot sicker than*

I think I am. I simply don't feel ready to be put out to pasture. I'm only fifty-nine years old."

What is wrong with this picture? These very nice people are up to their waists in a swamp of pain. When they most need and want to help one another, they are sinking in their tensions, frustrations, and fears—all because they are trying to hide the truth from one another. The irony, of course, is that no one is hiding anything very well. Henry Hinson knows his wife is hiding the bills; he even knows where they are. Maria knows her husband is miserable even though he hasn't said a word about it. And John, who has postponed his own life because he loves his parents so much, knows they're unhappy anyway: he sees his father, a vital man, languishing in the den all day, while his mother becomes thinner and spends several afternoons each week in bed with migraines. No one is talking about what's really going on, and everyone is quietly beginning to despair.

What can the Hinsons do differently *now* to repair their family? Now that you are dealing with heart disease, you face the same important choices: Will you let the stress of recovery pull you away from the people you love and who love you, or will you welcome the illness as a second-chance opportunity that draws you closer together?

FAMILY + FRIENDS = STRENGTH TO RECOVER

By understanding how support systems work—in sickness and in health—you can avoid the traps that many families fall into. The great news is that many people grow closer once the shock of heart illness abates. It's as though a brush with death reminds them of how important they are to one another.

I should mention here that when I talk about families, I don't mean only the man-and-woman-and-kids variety. To me, a family is a tribe, a clan, a cluster of human beings committed to one another's well-being. When I speak of family I mean support system and include under its umbrella straight couples and gay couples, with or without kids; single people living alone whose families are primarily networks of friends; older couples, none of whose family members live under their roof—in short, by family I mean those people around you, whether or not they live with you, whose presence gives your life meaning, and to whom you turn for friendship, love, care, and support.

If you are a single person living alone with heart disease, you must put extra effort into creating a nurturing family of friends to help you during your recovery and beyond. If you live alone, you are especially vulnerable to feelings of helplessness and frustration, and I urge you to resist the temptation to dig in, batten your emotional hatches, and try to recover alone. You might be able to do it, but the odds are against you. This is not the time to be a pioneer; you're not the little heart patient on the prairie. Go to the people closest to you, tell them you need them, and ask them for help. There's no weakness implicit in asking for help; on the contrary, it takes guts. If you're the kind of person who is comfortable asking for help, you're fortunate—and you'll hasten your recovery by doing it often. If you're the kind of person who would rather die than ask for help, you might get your wish if you don't reconsider your priorities. I assure you—preserving your pride is a feeble reward for diminishing the quality of your life, or even losing it.

Heart disease often redefines the health awareness of patients, their families, and even their friends. The time following a coronary event is a time to start showing how much you love one another and to stop doing the things that strain your relationships.

To build a healthy new attitude toward living with heart illness—in other words, to create and embrace your new normal—I tell my patients to take these four steps:

1. Start to see your family as a team.
2. Learn to recognize signs of relationship struggles.
3. Use my no-nonsense techniques to manage your recovery team.
4. Communicate.

A FAMILY IS A TEAM

Living with heart disease is similar to what happens when you toss a large rock into a small pond: the shock waves roll on and on, rippling through the lives of everyone close to the patient (as well as the patient him- or herself). Stress affects all members of a team. When illness strikes, your entire family and support group may feel the strain, making any and all members vulnerable to worry and struggle. Research shows that, when a heart patient is in the hospital, family members voice more fears about the future and the patient's health than the patient does.[1] And both heart patients and their families complain that health care providers don't pay enough attention to—or give adequate advice about—the issues family members face.[2]

When heart disease is diagnosed, patient and family members alike may experience sadness, anger, anxiety, grief, depression, and health worries where none existed before. I see this most often in my work with spouses of heart patients. It has been said that the patient may recover from the shock of heart disease but the mate may not. After all, it's the mate who sees the patient close to death, hooked up to tubing and electrical devices, inert and helpless. It's the mate who lies awake at night, listening to the breathing, worrying about what may happen next. It's the mate who, a full year later, sometimes continues to lie awake at three a.m., mentally rerunning those terrible hospital days over and over, long after the patient is feeling strong and vital again.

Sometimes, like Maria Hinson, a wife manipulates her family's dynamics and activities in a futile attempt to spin a cocoon around the patient. Or a husband may become a cheerleader, cultivating a bouncy, smiling facade that disguises his true feelings and prevents his wife from revealing hers. No wonder more than one third of heart patients' mates report significant emotional upset and loneliness,[3] and caregivers are at serious risk of developing stress-related health problems themselves, with wives seeming especially vulnerable.[4]

SIGNS THAT A FAMILY ISN'T COPING WELL

Caretaker burnout is just one sign that a family is struggling; there are many others. Here are ten common responses to heart disease—and examples of their verbal manifestations—that could indicate that your family isn't coping well. Some of them are typically expressed by patients, others by family members as well as patients.

1. **What it may sound like:**

   "I'll never be happy again, not the way I was before. People tell me I'll feel better soon, but they're wrong—I can't imagine feeling cheerful or hopeful again."

   What it may be:

   Depression.
   When you or someone you love is diagnosed with a serious illness, it's normal to be sad. Not only is it normal, it's extremely common: depending on the nature of the condition or surgery, between 40 and 75 percent of heart patients suffer periods of depression. Many, speaking of their

reactions to learning they had heart disease, have told me they were surprised at the intensity of their sadness, saying it felt like grief—which is exactly what it is.

Grief is an appropriate and healthy reaction to illness. You learn, suddenly and painfully, that your body is vulnerable and you must change the way you live your life if you want to hold on to it. It makes sense to feel that you've suffered a loss, because you have: the loss of the illusion of your immortality.

It takes time for the meaning of this loss to sink in, both for heart patients and the people who care about them. A grieving person may weep easily and often, act irritable, be unable to sleep, and worry about whether life will ever feel good again. These behaviors usually pass after a few months as people realize they can live with heart disease, and, indeed, that they want to. The will to survive is supplanted by the decision to thrive, and patient and support system start moving toward rehabilitation.

But sometimes the grief doesn't abate. Sometimes a patient or family member simply cannot get beyond bereavement and falls into depression—a condition that paralyzes everyone concerned and inhibits recovery. If a person is still deeply upset more than three months after heart disease is diagnosed, he or she may be clinically depressed.

Depression is a serious medical condition and should be treated by a medical or mental health professional. It is important to deal with depression because it drives some people into complete emotional and physical shutdown: they can no longer cry, and other emotional responses flatten out; they lose track of time, sometimes even forgetting to eat; their zest for life dwindles so that nothing can spark their interest; and nothing that anyone says can make it any better. Pep talks, motivational tapes, lectures on positive thinking, and friendly exhortations to get out there and pull yourself up by your bootstraps will not lift you or anyone else out of a serious depression.

What you can do:

Get help. The good news is that not only can we treat depression, we can cure it. Millions—that's right, *millions*—of people vanquish depression every year with the right combination of counseling and medication. Of course, the right combination is the combination that's right for you, and you may need help to figure out what that combination is. If you or any member of your family still feels profoundly sad for more than three months after heart disease is diagnosed, get professional help. (One thing you can do right away is turn to Chapter 7, which deals with depression in greater detail.)

2. What it may sound like:

Patient: "This is *not* happening to me. I don't want to deal with it, I don't want to learn about it, I don't want to hear about it."

What it may be:

Denial of the symptoms and the diagnosis.

Some patients and family members cannot bear to acknowledge that heart disease has invaded their lives, so they deny the symptoms, the diagnosis, or both. This usually happens because they're too frightened to think rationally about what the illness really means. They act as though the cardiac episode is either a fluke or hasn't happened at all, preventing anyone from adjusting to the situation. Women are more likely than men to deny the severity of their symptoms, mistakenly believing that heart illness is a man's disease and waiting longer before getting to a hospital for treatment.

One family I treated insisted on referring to their father's angina as upset stomach. Another family changed doctors five times until they found one who would play along, gloss over the symptoms, and prescribe Pepto-Bismol instead of a bypass. I've lost count of the patients who chose to sleep through the wake-up call of their diagnosis, saying "High blood pressure runs in my family, and no one under sixty-five has ever died of it. Trust me—it's nothing to worry about."

As I mentioned earlier, denial might lessen your anxiety in the short run, but it will cause problems if you use it as a long-term coping strategy. Denial interferes with a family's ability to work as a team and increases the likelihood that the patient will wait too long before seeking treatment if symptoms return.

What you can do:

Be prepared—know the symptoms of heart disease when you feel them. If you understand what you're feeling (or seeing, if you're a family member), you'll be better able to remain calm and think rationally and less tempted to deny what's happening. Cardiologists like to say that time is muscle, and they're right: every moment you sit around wondering whether your chest pain is bad enough to warrant a trip to the emergency room is precious time that could allow further damage to your heart muscle. With some planning, you can learn to recognize the symptoms of a cardiac emergency and avert the temptation to deny it.

Signs and Symptoms of Heart Disease [5]

You might be having a heart attack if:

- Your chest pain begins and builds in intensity over a minute or two and is located toward the center rather than left side of the chest.

- The pain lasts for at least twenty minutes and is not relieved when you rest or change positions.

- The pain usually feels like pressure or heaviness and ranges from mild to severe.

- The pain radiates up into your jaw or down your back or left arm.

- You experience nausea, shortness of breath, or a sense of impending doom.

- You experience subtle but atypical symptoms such as indigestion or difficulty breathing (women are especially prone to such symptoms).

If you have diabetes, pay particular attention to any chest discomfort you may feel, because your body is susceptible to misinterpreting pain messages.

See your doctor if you experience:

- Chest pain that is unusual for you

- Frequent or severe palpitations

- Unexplained fainting

- Severe shortness of breath

- Overwhelming fatigue

- Bodily swelling

If you have chest pain for more than fifteen minutes, get to a hospital. Don't worry about bothering the doctors if it turns out to be heartburn—doctors would rather diagnose a bad case of indigestion than sign a death certificate. Do yourself a favor—bother the folks in the emergency room and save your own life (or someone else's).

Another thing you can do is challenge denial when and where you find it. If you're the patient and the person you live with keeps serving French fries with dinner, gently remind him or her that oily foods are hazardous to your health (but do wait until the company leaves). If your father resumes smoking two packs of cigarettes a week after his bypass surgery, sit down, look him in the eye, and tell him how hard it is for you to watch him harming himself. These conversations are awkward at best and painful at worst, but if you don't challenge denial, you're participating in it.

3. **What it may sound like:**

"Damn right I'm angry—I've got every right to be!"

What it may be:

Chronic, mismanaged anger and hostility.

Many people are angry long before heart disease disrupts their lives. When these folks learn they have heart disease, they grow even more hostile, losing emotional control over even minor annoyances. A ten-minute wait in a supermarket line or misplaced car keys can set such a person off on a nasty verbal assault, to the astonishment of everyone around him. This type of person always had a low anger threshold; heart disease merely lowered the bar.

Other people, however, are surprised at their newfound hostility. They find themselves feeling irritable and moody, throwing temper tantrums for the first time since they were three, and snapping at the people who are trying hardest to help them. This often means they are trapped in the anger stage of grief, unable to get past the resentment that this had to happen to them. It's the same feeling we had when we were little and thought we'd been punished unjustly; we kicked and screamed about how unfair it all was, blaming Mom and Dad for our misfortune. But now we're adults, and our rational side tells us we can't blame our parents (at least not *only* our parents), so instead we blame anyone and everyone who ticks us off, which doesn't take much.

What you can do:

First: When you feel your anger rising, stop, inhale deeply through your nose, and exhale slowly through your mouth. Then, do it again. In other words, take a deep breath . . . and then another, and another. This will relax you and lower your heart rate. You can do it anywhere—in line at the market so you don't bawl out the checkout kid who's taking so long, or at home so you don't shout at your mate for using your car and losing your keys (or after your mate shouts at *you* for losing the keys). No one will know what you're doing, and everyone will benefit, especially you.

Second: as you start to relax, ask yourself, "If I weren't this angry, what *else* might I be feeling?" Anger often marks the flash point of other upsetting feelings, especially those that may be frightening to acknowledge. Families may use anger to mask feelings of vulnerability such as fear, sadness, awkwardness, or insecurity. Anger is more familiar than these other emotions and less threatening to experience.

Imagine you're that person in line at the market, stewing because you're in the express lane—ten items only—and the guy in front of you obviously has thirteen, one of which requires a price check. You're all tuned up because the sign clearly states the ten-item rule, yet this inconsiderate creep ignores the sign, breaks the rule, and holds up the whole line. *You* read the sign and *you* obeyed the rule—why should you be made to wait?

What should you do now? Right. Stop. Take a deep breath, and then another, and another. As your heart rate goes down and you return to your senses, ask yourself, "If I weren't so angry, what else might I be feeling?" While this man's lack of consideration is annoying, it's possible that what you're really angry about is that you followed all the rules—you quit smoking, you're only ten pounds overweight, you don't eat fries as often as your buddies do—and you got heart disease anyway. Maybe you're angry at all those people who *don't* follow the rules—who smoke, weigh too much, eat fries (and hog the express checkout line)—who seem to be just fine.

Recognizing the source of your hostility is the first step to managing it. (For more steps, see Chapter 8.)

4. What it may sound like:

"Let's live as much as we can as fast as we can."

What it may be:

Frantic flights into activity (and away from reality).

Some people see heart disease as a death sentence and start flying frantically from one activity to another. They are anxious about how much time they have left and want to cram as much living as possible into their remaining days.

There's nothing wrong with deciding to live each day as if it's your last; in fact, it's a good thing to do because it reminds you of how precious life really is. The problem is, busier doesn't always mean happier; when living is fueled by desperation, joy is seldom part of it.

The frantic flight syndrome may be hard to recognize at first. A heart patient who flies from the shopping mall to volunteer at a Red Cross blood drive, then on to read to her granddaughter's class and then on to her bridge club may look like a positive-thinking dynamo; in reality, she's merely hyperactive. She is taking physical health risks by not allowing herself sufficient time to rest and emotional health risks by substituting fleeting contact with others for meaningful connection. She's not focusing on anything enough to experience it fully; she's focusing obsessively on action, not the content of her actions. Sometimes the patient hurls him- or herself into exhausting bouts of activity; other times, the family spins into tornado mode, and at its center is the patient, wondering why every moment is so charged with urgency.

What you can do:

Slow down, sit still, and take stock. Doing more doesn't mean you're living more—it means you're rushing more, bustling more, valuing the quantity of your actions over the quality of your interactions.

Have the fortitude to sit still—it takes courage to sit tight when everything in you cries out to run away. Will yourself to quiet your mind and listen to your inner voice. What are you afraid of? Are your fears rooted in reality or the lush soil of Fantasy Island? Remember: most people with heart illness who take reasonable care of themselves live to a ripe old age. This means *you*. Learn about your condition, and find out what taking care of yourself means as you define and create your new normal.

Don't let fear of loss push you away from others. Some families fling themselves into frantic action because they dread growing even more attached to the patient than they already are. They're afraid their loved one will die, and they begin preparing themselves for the loss when the illness first hits. The irony is that these families are still sometimes keep-ing their distance while the patient outlives everyone else.

If you care about a heart patient, don't retreat from the connection, and don't be satisfied with merely maintaining it. Instead, deepen it. Work on *being* together instead of merely doing things together. If you've been watching videos every night, go out to dinner instead and have a conversation. Talk. Listen. Connect.

5. **What it may sound like:**

"This is so enormous, so overwhelming. I think we should just let nature take its course."

What it may be:

Passive acceptance of the illness.

Heart disease is a second-chance illness, but you get that second chance only if you wake up and start living better. Some people simply cannot cope with illness, so they passively accept their fate and refuse to participate in either their own recovery or that of their loved one. They won't attend classes on heart-healthy living, won't go to cardiac rehabili-tation, won't see a therapist. Some patients even fail to show up for their follow-up appointments with the cardiologist.

What you can do:

Don't passively accept your fate—actively create your future. Fear of the unknown—and the heart is a classic symbol of that which is unknowable about us—is often lurking beneath passive acceptance of heart disease. Peo-ple are so afraid of what they'll find out, they refuse to learn what will make them well. What a shame—nine times out of ten, the truth about heart dis-ease is far less frightening than not getting help. Get yourself into a cardiac rehabilitation program; show up for your doctor's appointments; learn about heart-healthy foods and how to prepare them, and make sure you start eat-ing them (and get the people around you to eat better, too).

6. **What it may sound like:**

"I don't want to burden you with my problems. You've been through enough already."

What it may be:

Protective buffering.

Maria Hinson's antistress strategy, deployed with such damaging results, is an example of protective buffering. People who use this strategy usually do so out of concern for others and think they are being helpful; in reality, too much of this kind of protection can actually hurt heart patients, their mates, family members, and friends.

A recent study tracked forty-three male heart attack survivors. The patients and their wives were interviewed a month after coming home from the hospital, and again six months later. At the time of either interview, couples who engaged in protective buffering revealed higher levels of distress than couples who didn't. And it didn't matter who was doing the buffering: when either patient or spouse tried to hide the truth from the other, neither person adjusted well.[6]

What you can do:

Stop trying to control everyone's life by de-emphasizing yours. It is enormously frustrating to be around someone who always acts as if she or he is the least important person in the room. It makes other people feel selfish for admitting they have needs.

Stop hiding and tell the truth. If you're the patient, don't pretend you're fine, dandy, and ready to run the New York Marathon. Hardly anyone can run the New York Marathon, including some of the people who try. Be honest with yourself and others.

As you recover, celebrate your advances and acknowledge your vulnerabilities. If you get tired after being on your feet for two hours, don't beg off when your daughter invites you to go to the mall; instead, ask her to make the shopping expedition a brief one. Then put on your walking shoes and go.

If you're not the patient, the same goes for you: shed your cloak of self-denial and admit that you have needs, too.

7. **What it may sound like:**

"I know you're not feeling great, but I feel lousy too."

(Variations: "I'm more tired than you are"; "My headache's worse than yours"; "I'm recovering from major surgery and you aren't"; etc.)

What it may be:

Competing for sympathy.

You know it's time for a reality check if you find yourself competing in a suffering sweepstakes. The only prize here is the booby prize, and you'll get it if you're trying to get your needs met by complaining instead of communicating.

This attitude is the opposite of the last one: instead of negating your needs, you inflate them in the hope that others will realize how unhappy you are. This syndrome usually develops when a person feels that his or her needs are being ignored and lacks the confidence to say so.

What you can do:

Quit whining and communicate. When you feel the need to express how bad you feel or how unhappy you are, ask yourself: Are you trying to communicate a feeling or complain about it? Are you trying to explain yourself to another human being or make that person understand that your pain is worse than his (or hers)?

8. What it may sound like:

"For years I've been trying to get you to listen to me, but you never did. Now maybe you'll admit that I was right all along."
(Also known as "It's my way or the highway.")

What it may be:

Using the illness to wield power in a relationship.

Some people use illness to exert power over others—mates, children, parents, and friends—whom they've found difficult to influence in the past. The illness becomes the arena in which unresolved family conflicts are battled. This coping strategy is just as likely to be used by family members as by patients. A grown son whose father suffers a serious heart attack says, "Well, Dad, now that you've nearly killed yourself with cigarettes, maybe you'll finally listen to me. My whole life, you've never heard a word I've said—maybe now you will." The father might respond with "If I've never heard a word you've said, it's because you've never treated me the way a son should treat a father. I worked my whole life so you could go to good schools and wear hundred-dollar sneakers. *I'm* the one who's sick, so *I'm* the one who gets to call the shots around here."

Both men think they're arguing about how to best take care of Dad, but they're really fighting about issues that go back twenty-five years and have nothing to do with improving anyone's health.

What you can do:

Resist the urge to use the illness as a weapon in a relationship struggle. There's nothing more satisfying than hurling a well-deserved I-told-you-so—and few things more likely to ignite a fight. Your objective now is to adjust to living with heart disease and create a new normal, not to prove who is right and who was wronged.

Try to resolve your differences by talking things out—advice that's easier for me to give than for you to do. Still, it is possible to use words to work out your differences. To help you do it, I've included some communication techniques in the next chapter. If those don't help, get counseling. Don't wait until it's too late; escalating family hostility creates health risks for both recovering cardiac patients and the people around them.

9. What it may sound like:

"We can't agree on *anything* anymore."

What it may be:

Conflicting coping strategies.

Tensions often develop between family members about what heart disease means and what they should do about it. (Friends may also find themselves embroiled in disagreements with the patient and family about how to interpret the new normal.) While each person's coping strategy might have merit, having five or six different ones will likely breed conflict. The person who cooks for the family might start serving dry grilled chicken three nights a week and find four glum faces at the table. Or a friend might cope by choosing not to take the heart attack seriously and lighting up a cigarette the way she always does when she arrives.

What you can do:

From time to time, sit down and talk about what each of you is going through. Be honest and clear about what you think is happening and how you would like to handle it. Avoid problems by making sure that you and your loved ones are approaching rehabilitation in similar ways.

10. **What it may sound like:**

"What's gotten into the kids lately?"

What it may be:

Children (or teenagers or grandchildren) in distress.

If heart disease is frightening for adults, it can be even more terrifying for children. Those little eyes and ears often interpret the events surrounding an illness in desperate ways. Even the most compassionate adults sometimes forget that children, teenagers, and grandchildren struggle mightily with the emotional turmoil heart illness can bring. Even children who seem to be coping well may be hiding a tornado of emotion, which can lead to psychological, emotional, and academic difficulties.

Josh and Helen had to deal with the reactions of their daughters, Lucy and Karen, after Josh's heart attack. A recent conversation with the family illustrates what they went through:

> HELEN: It all happened so fast. Josh was in and out of the hospital before we realized what the illness really meant. The girls asked questions, and we answered as best we could. But I don't think they understood the seriousness of what had happened.
>
> The hardest part was when Josh went back into the hospital four months later with chest pains. We spent two weeks trying to figure out what to do. Finally, the doctors told us that Josh needed open-heart surgery. When the children visited him in the recovery room, they had a difficult time. I'll never forget when they first saw him, hooked up to

oxygen and intravenous lines. He looked so pale, so frail, so not like the daddy they knew. That was hard on them.

LUCY (AGE NINE): It was really scary seeing Dad that first time—he looked a little dead to me. But then I saw him breathing, and I knew he was alive, just very weak. Later, I'd listen when the doctors would talk to my mom and dad. I couldn't understand everything they were saying, but I did understand a little, and that helped.

KAREN (AGE SIX): My mommy helped me, and my daddy, too, when he could. They helped me not to worry. But I still worry about Mommy. She cries sometimes at night when I'm in bed. I'm afraid she'll worry too much and then she'll get sick, too.

Lucy and Karen are lucky: They have loving, concerned parents who see them as separate beings struggling, each in her own way, with their father's illness. They also have learned that it is safe to express their fears within the family. Talking about what scares them has helped these youngsters enjoy a normal childhood despite the family's changed circumstances.

But when illness comes, even children in loving families may show delayed stress reactions. When a child represses inner turmoil, various problems may develop, depending on the child's age:

- Declining grades at school
- Eating or sleeping disorders
- Frequent or recurring nightmares, or both
- Outbursts of temper
- Vague or persistent physical problems
- Fears of being alone with the patient
- Clinging to parents and other comforting adults
- Excessive fatigue
- A tendency to withdraw from people and situations
- Drug or alcohol use
- Trying too hard to please or "be good"
- Rebellious behaviors
- Inability or refusal to discuss problems, especially feelings about the illness

If your children or grandchildren are showing signs of struggle, don't feel guilty and don't despair. You can help them cope with the illness by taking these steps:

- Find out if they're worrying.

- Talk about the situation. If you're the patient, tell the kids how you're doing.

- Ask if they have questions, and try to reassure them with your answers.

- Give them information that gives them hope. They listen more than they let on.

- Admit you don't know all the answers. If a child asks if you're going to need another operation and even your cardiologist doesn't know yet, say, "I wonder about that myself. I'm not sure, but I have a very good doctor who's taking good care of me." Reassure the child that you're getting good medical care.

- Give children permission to talk about their fears. If you're unable to calm their worries, consider taking them to a therapist.

- Tell school counselors about the illness. They in turn can ask the children's teachers to watch for uncharacteristic behaviors.

- Make sure the children understand that they had nothing to do with causing your illness. Young children are especially likely to imagine that something they have said or done may have brought on your condition.

- Talk openly and frequently about your recovery and rehabilitation. An aura of secrecy isolates heart patients from their families, and family members and friends from one another.

I've never met a family that experienced all ten of these struggles—at least not all at once. In fact, many families I know have experienced *none* of these struggles. If you are among the lucky ones, great! And, if your family is experiencing some of these struggles, you're still among the lucky ones—you're here, and you're dealing with your illness.

Don't let the struggles cast a shadow over the hard-won progress you've made. Be grateful for the support you're getting, and don't keep it to yourself. Let every member of your family and support system know that you appreciate their teamwork, and acknowledge that you know it isn't always easy. And just in case it isn't easy for you to talk to the people you're closest to, you'll find some pointers in Chapter 4.

Chapter Four ·

NO-NONSENSE TECHNIQUES FOR MANAGING YOUR RECOVERY TEAM

(or How to Talk to Your Family Without Getting Them All Ticked Off)

Why include a chapter on family communication techniques? Because the people we're closest to are not always equipped to help us the way we need to be helped. Speaking the heart's deepest feelings can tie the tongue of the most eloquent person.

When heart illness descends, a family may feel gripped in a vise of anxiety and stress. And when people are stressed, they sometimes do things that hurt rather than help one another cope with the illness. In my practice, I often see family members misinterpret one another's efforts to help. Reminding the patient to skip the fries comes across as pestering; an invitation to go for a walk sounds like an accusation of laziness. Your family and support network can become polarized, with the patient at one end and family members, relatives, and friends at the other, glaring at one another across a minefield of good intentions.

You must work with your family and friends to recruit a recovery team that supports each of you. As you develop your team, remember that different people have different strengths and should not be expected to perform with equal ability. Don't expect your cynical son to be a cheerleader; it's not in his nature. Instead, suggest he research your HMO's cardiologists to learn which one's training and personal style are best suited to you. His natural skepticism will increase your chances of choosing the right physician. Likewise, don't expect your partner to drag you out walking if she hates to exercise; ask a friend to walk with you instead. It would be ideal if friends and family members would renovate their personalities to accommodate your recovery from heart illness, but that's not how people are. People do modify their behaviors, but they usually stop short of a personality overhaul.

From your family's point of view, it would be easier if you'd had an epiphany along with the heart attack and followed through with any promises you made in the CCU to give up smoking, pizza, and six-packs—but that usually doesn't happen. It's not human nature to reverse a lifetime of habits instantly, so be patient—both with yourself and with the people on your recovery team.

Remember—no one does this perfectly; every family coping with heart illness has disagreements and goes through some tense times. But if you all work at it, you'll start to see one another as parts of a whole, as members of a team, and your teamwork will improve.

Here are some tips to give your family and friends on how to enhance teamwork:

1. **Talk with one another so that all team members understand your condition and what must be done to cope with it.** Discuss your condition honestly and openly; neither minimize nor exaggerate the dangers or risks. Secrecy, not openness, feeds fear.

2. **Remember that coping with illness is a group endeavor, a family affair.** Any member of the team may show signs of stress—it's not always the person with the heaviest workload or the shakiest coping skills. Sometimes the toughest cookie is the first to crumble, while the shrinking violet blossoms into a bulwark of strength.

    Sharpen your awareness of the people around you. Look for symptoms of coping problems, and ask family members how they're feeling about life in general and the illness in particular. Stay on the lookout past the first few months; the first couple of years after the diagnosis is when caregivers are in greatest danger of burning out.

3. **Make a habit of telling one another that you believe in one another.** Show that you appreciate each member of your recovery team—close family members, relatives, friends, even colleagues—by putting your gratitude into words, and encourage one another to bear up under the strain. We all need praise and reminders that we are making progress.

4. **From time to time, ask your team members if they're getting the right kind of support (and let them know if you're not receiving it from them).** People change; the wife who insists she's got everything under control one week may be trembling with fatigue the next. Likewise, the patient who needs a pep talk on Monday may be giving one on Wednesday. The challenges of adjusting to heart illness vary, and as they do, the team must adjust the kind of support it offers.

5. **Aggressively seek and share information related to heart-healthy living. Medical breakthroughs happen every day, and one of them might save your life.** Just two weeks after this book first appeared, the Food and Drug Administration approved a device that could save millions of lives: a new, drug-coated stent—a small, metal mesh tube that gets inserted in an artery to keep it open after angioplasty. This was a breakthrough because, until then, the artery would often reclog as plaque adhered to the stent (a process doctors refer to as restenosis). But the new stent is coated with a chemical (sirolimus, also known as rapamycin) that prevents plaque from adhering to it, keeping the artery open and *profoundly improving the prospects for people with clogged arteries.*[1] In another development, researchers have found that C-reactive protein, a substance secreted by the liver and detected with a simple blood test, may predict heart illness even more accurately than do raised cholesterol levels (see box on p. 68). Hearing about breakthroughs like these will boost your morale (and possibly your life expectancy if your arteries are clogged).

If you're already tuned in to health-related broadcasts and publications, fine-tune your receiver for information on heart health (if you're *not* on a heart-healthy wavelength, tune in *now*). If your team members are well connected to the Internet and other information sources, ask them to scour different areas for information. If someone follows current events by reading newspapers on-line, have her regularly check the health sections of several major dailies for heart-related stories. If another team member subscribes to health magazines and newsletters, have him clip all articles that might be relevant, including, for instance, stories on reducing stress and depression, as well as those dealing directly with heart illness.

If you're a family member of someone with heart illness, you should also orient yourself toward learning about cardiac health. If there's a story in the newspaper about the benefits of cardiovascular exercise to heart patients, pass it on to the patient. If you learn your favorite talk-show host is doing a program on low-cholesterol cooking, tape it and present it to the family chef. If you're the only one in the patient's orbit who's hooked up to the Web, surf the American Heart Association site and others listed in the Resources section for breaking news on heart disease.

In short: When you learn something that might benefit the heart patient in your life (or anyone you care about), don't assume he or she already knows about it. Instead, take responsibility for spreading the news, and urge others on the team to do the same.

6. **Understand and accept that everyone changes at his or her own pace.** As a heart patient, you are not suffering from a contagious condition, and your eagerness to change your way of life may not be contagious, either. If you assume that everyone shares your enthusiasm, you risk alienating, not motivating, the very people you long to convert. Instead,

quietly go about your business, abandoning unhealthy behaviors, embracing healthy ones, and setting a good example.

7. **Work to keep intimacy alive.** If you have heart disease, intimacy isn't a luxury, it's a necessity. Intimacy does more than make you feel good; *intimacy can actually make your heart healthier.*[2] (I am not referring to sex; I'll talk about sexual intimacy and heart illness in Chapter 9.)

By intimacy, I mean staying lovingly in communication with your mate, immediate family, relatives, and friends. Intimate relationships diminish the effects of stress by making us feel less alone and reminding us that others will take up some of our burden. Intimacy thrives on the quality, not the quantity, of your relationships: you can be married with

---

FOR WOMEN, MARRIAGE IS NOT ENOUGH (HAPPINESS HELPS)

While it's true that a vigorous, loving primary relationship benefits both men and women, it is also true that the quality of a female heart patient's primary relationship has a greater impact on how long she will live than that of a male heart patient. Not only that: for a woman recovering from heart illness, it is marital stress, not work stress, that predicts more reliably whether she will have another cardiac event or even die.[3]

---

three kids and sadly lacking in intimacy; likewise, you can live alone and be intimately connected to a caring circle of friends.

Intimacy doesn't nudge its own way into your life and curl up in your lap—it comes only when you pursue it with energy and openness (yes, you have to work at it). Part of the work involves forgiving one another for past hurts and committing yourselves to learning to get along better. If you're holding on to a grudge that's older than that chunk of cheese at the back of the refrigerator, it's time to chuck out both of them. Clinging to resentment pushes you away from others and kills intimacy.

Perhaps the most crucial element in your recovery is that you maintain a robust friendship with each family member. Can you listen—*really* listen—when your children come to you with their fears, or do you feel obligated to deliver an I'm-fine-everything's-dandy monologue? Are you a good friend to your mate, or are you merely married? Intimacy grows when you let your loved ones know you cherish them. Here are suggestions for things you can say to one another *at least once every day:*

- "I'm so proud of you."

- "I admire you for being able to manage so many responsibilities." (Or being such a good big brother, being so helpful to your parents, acting so gracious when the house is full of people and all you want to do is sleep, and so on.)

- "I was bragging about you today. Here's what I said: '_____.'" (Fill in the blank with a rip-roaring compliment.)

- "You are one of my all-time favorite people." (And then say why.)

- "I love you." (Short, simple, effective.)

- "I was thinking today about all the things you mean to this family. I really do appreciate you."

- "I don't know what I'd do without you."

If you want to cultivate and maintain intimacy, **communicate!**

If statements like these are ricocheting around your household, your family is harboring a cardiac risk factor—poor communication:

- "She never listens to me."

- "I have no idea what you're talking about."

- "I'm not sure how my husband is doing; he never talks about his feelings."

- "Could we turn off the TV while we discuss this?"

- "How am I supposed to know what you want if you never tell me?"

Poor communication is not only one of the major stumbling blocks in relationships, it also can damage your heart. A person whose family is roiled by conflict or dampened by lack of closeness is more likely to experience an increase in blood pressure and heart rate, a higher level of stress hormones, and an imbalance in the autoimmune system.[4]
These next two tips are for family members.

8. **Adopt a "no martyrs, no spectators" policy.** No one person should have to shoulder all the stress that comes with the caretaking role. Each of you must shoulder your share of the burden, and dispense a commensurate dose of encouragement and support. In addition, each of you needs to feel necessary; no one likes to sit in the dugout while the rest of the team is hitting home runs.

9. **Allow the patient to be a source of strength.** We all need to be needed, which means that team members should sometimes turn to the heart patient

for support. Don't treat the patient as if he or she is at death's door. The patient is very much alive and eventually will be well. Keep the patient working with the team, and acknowledge his or her strength and spirit.

10. **Whether you're the patient or a family member, bear in mind the following tips** when dealing with relatives, friends, and everyone on the recovery team: [5]

Do's and Don'ts for Showing Support to Loved Ones (and Liked Ones, Too)

DO:	DON'T:
Remind	Nag
Participate	Shun
Discuss	Stay silent
Compliment	Criticize
Notice	Ignore
Encourage	Complain
Suggest	Lecture
Share information	Compete
Respect your differences	Expect to be the same
Listen	Talk incessantly
Reassure	Dwell on the worst-case scenario
Empathize	Insist on acting cheery
Sympathize	Pretend you know what it feels like if you don't
Cherish	Take for granted

TALK TO ONE ANOTHER

Cardiac families often settle into strained communication patterns because they fear that discussing emotional issues will be hazardous to the patient's health. This misperception is a common one. Remember that family conflict is a normal part of life and is not dangerous to your health; *mismanaged* conflict is. Effective communication between patient and family and among family members themselves, as well as among all members of the team, is an important part of cardiac recovery.

Here are some suggestions for communicating more effectively:

• **Develop a communication habit.** People in healthy relationships make time to talk and air their differences as conflicts evolve, rather than let tensions accumulate. This involves creating situations that are conducive to communication. One couple I know walks together before breakfast on Mondays, Wednesdays, and Fridays; if it's raining, they reschedule for the weekend. Another family sits down in the den for a thirty-minute chat after Sunday dinner—with the television off—because there are three children with different schedules and that's the one day everyone can usually attend. During hectic times, you can visit in ten-minute spurts before moving on to your next activity; one father I know talks with his daughter as he drives her to field hockey practice. It doesn't matter what you do; what matters is that you do something regularly that creates a safe forum in which to communicate.

- **Be a good listener.** Listening, not speaking, is the most important communication skill. Being a good listener is challenging because you must control your impulse to respond immediately and wait until it's appropriate to do so. It also means paying attention to more than a person's words and noticing nonverbal behaviors as well.

  When you converse with someone, it's important to concentrate on two things: the speaker's message and the feelings behind the message. Take note of the speaker's tone of voice and body language as well as the words. Does he or she seem upset, afraid, or angry? If she swears that she's not annoyed but her arms are crossed over her chest and her eyes are slightly narrowed, she may be very much annoyed but reluctant to say so. If he claims he's doing just fine in a loud, cheerful voice but can't meet your eyes when he says so, he may not be doing as fine as his words would indicate.

  Being a good listener takes practice. You have to repress the urge to interrupt and discipline yourself to really concentrate—even when you're tired, grouchy, or preoccupied with your own troubles. All of us have daydreamed through conversations that deserved more of our attention, realizing later that we missed something significant because we were too busy listening to our own thoughts rather than the words of the person speaking to us. But don't despair: every day offers you numerous opportunities to improve your listening skills.

- **Let other people know you hear them, on all levels.** A simple "I hear you" or "You know, that makes sense" might do. Nodding your head and murmuring "Um-hm" a few times while another person is speaking will also convey that you are listening. And there's nothing like eye contact to let the other person know you're paying attention.

  Sometimes, though, people will feel heard only if you let them know that you understand both *what* they are saying and *why* they are saying it. For example, if your mate has just chided you for not phoning in when you were out all afternoon, you might start your response by restating the problem so that she or he knows you were, indeed, listening. Here's an example:

FAMILY MEMBER: "You know, I was worried sick for the last two hours. How am I supposed to know you're all right and not in the emergency room somewhere?"

PATIENT: "Mmm . . . I guess you get frightened if I'm out for a while and you don't hear from me. Is that right?"

FAMILY MEMBER: "Yes, that's right! I just get so worried when you're away from me and I don't know where you are."

PATIENT: "All right, I can understand that; I'm sorry I scared you. Next time, I'll call you if I'm going to be out longer than I said I would."

Resist the temptation to defend yourself or respond angrily, even if you've been dealt with in an angry way. Remember the source of the anger is love, after all, and concern for your welfare.

Finally, let the speaker know that you empathize with him or her: "Gee— I'm sorry that I upset you so much. I didn't mean to. If I were in your place, I'd feel the same way, and I'd probably be even angrier than you are. I know that you're concerned about me, and I do appreciate it. Thanks."

• **If you don't understand someone's response to an issue, ask for more information.** Sometimes a person insists that something you've done has caused him or her distress or harm, and you don't have the slightest idea of what you did. Again, resist the temptation to defend yourself against the attack, and strive instead to understand the other person's point of view, even when you think he or she is being unreasonable, as follows:

PATIENT: "Where did you go? I've been calling your name for five minutes! Where were you?"

YOU: "I've been right here. I just walked outside to get the mail."

PATIENT: "How are you supposed to hear me if you go outside? What if something happens? How will you know?"

YOU: "I'll know because I come right back. Please—help me understand. Why is this so frightening for you? What are you afraid might happen?"

If you still don't understand the person's reaction, ask for more specific information: "Could you be more specific? I want to understand this from your point of view."

• **Express confidence in the future.** When you're in the midst of sorting out a misunderstanding, remind yourself (and the person you're struggling with) that things will go smoother in the future once you get through the present awkwardness. In a way that neither blames nor disparages, describe what you learned about the person and the situation, and express your expectation that this knowledge will help you handle things better from now on. You might say, "I don't like it when we squabble, but I did learn something important: I learned that you feel most secure when you know where I am. I'll keep this in mind from now on. In the meantime, I want you to know that I love you, and I know we can work this through as long as we keep talking to each other, even when it's hard."

- **Make your needs known.** Start by first asking if the other person is willing to listen: "There's something I'd like to discuss with you. Are you open to hearing me out?" Next, use "I" messages to express what's on your mind, taking care to state what *you* feel, need, or want. Do not talk about what the other person is doing or not doing—in other words, avoid expressing your feelings in terms that blame the other person for your troubles.

Here are some blaming messages and some more effective "I" messages to use instead:

BLAMING MESSAGE: "I'm sick and tired of the way you're always preaching to me about what I should eat!"

"I" MESSAGE: "I'd like to talk with you about something. I know that you're concerned about my health, but I feel irritated when you comment on what I eat, especially in front of others. I'd be happier if you'd let me handle my diet."

BLAMING MESSAGE: "You're always nagging me about taking my medicine. If you'd just give me a chance, I'd take it on my own!"

"I" MESSAGE: "I know how much you care about me, but when you remind me to take my medicine so frequently, I feel that you're treating me like a child. I'd feel better if you'd trust me to manage my medication."

When expressing yourself, use phrases such as "I feel . . . ," "In my opinion . . . ," and "I'm afraid that . . ." Avoid phrases such as "You always . . . ," "You never . . . ," and "I can't believe that you . . ." You can't go wrong if you talk about what *you* think and feel. Once you start talking about what others think and feel, you're on shaky ground, even when you're right.

- **When you ask for what you want, be specific.** It may be difficult to tell others what you want of them, so you may slide into vague requests that sound less demanding than what you'd actually like. As time passes and your needs go unmet, you'll start to feel lonely and resentful.

It's best to be direct. When you broach the subject of what you'd like someone to do for you, take a deep breath, look the person in the eye, and say exactly what you'd like him or her to do (or not do, as the case may be). The more specific you are, the more likely it is that the person will fulfill your request.

Here are some examples of vague (ineffective) and specific (effective) ways of expressing yourself:

VAGUE: "I don't imagine you're planning on taking a walk today?"

SPECIFIC: "It would mean a lot to me if you'd go walking with me today. How about it?"

VAGUE: "It would be good if we could eat healthier meals sometimes."

SPECIFIC: "I'd prefer not to take in Chinese food tonight, if that's okay with you. It's cooked with a lot of oil and salt, and eating it several times a week isn't good for me."

And if you're the caretaker, here's one for you:

VAGUE: "Do you think you'll be wanting me to come back later tonight?"

SPECIFIC: "A friend's invited me to join him for dinner tonight, and I'd like to go. Will you be all right on your own, or shall I call Ellen and see if she can come over?"

- **Learn to say no.** Making your needs known sometimes means having to say no to friends and loved ones, especially when they make you offers you'd just as soon refuse.

Imagine that you live alone and your neighbor Mike shows up three nights a week with an armful of videos, invites himself in, and settles down for an evening of movie musical classics, which you could easily live without. He means well and you don't want to offend him, so you open the door and resign yourself to yet another screening of *Oklahoma!* Before long, you realize that you and Ado Annie have a lot in common as she lilts into the all-too-familiar strains of "I Cain't Say No."

Well, you *can* say no, and you must learn to do it. Rather than suffer silently and feel resentful, learn to say no—diplomatically and firmly. Next time Mike shows up, invite him into the foyer, smile, look him in the eye, and say, "Mike, it is so kind of you to come by. Your support means a lot to me, but I'm taking a break from movies and catching up on my reading. May I give you a call when I'm back in a Hollywood frame of mind?" Unless Mike is completely out of touch, he'll get the message and depart quickly.

Remember that it helps to be specific. And let the other person know that, even though you're declining the offer, you know he or she is trying to help. Here's another example of how to say no tactfully:

FAMILY MEMBER: "It's so beautiful out today! Let's not forget to go for a walk."

PATIENT: "You're right, the weather is perfect for a walk. But I'm not feeling up to it today. Could we maybe sit on the deck and read the newspaper instead?"

- **During a conflict, deal with one topic at a time.** It is natural during a family discussion—especially the heated kind—for unfinished business to surface. Trying to resolve multiple issues in a single discussion leaves you frustrated because nothing gets resolved. Instead, take the position that an important issue deserves its own discussion; then stick to that issue until it is resolved. Save other important issues for future discussions.

- **Avoid participating in communication triangles.** When tension mounts between two people, it's common for each to focus on a third person rather than deal with each other. This never works out well, especially for the person in the middle. Here are some ways to avoid ending up there:
  - Stay calm and emotionally neutral when dealing with feuding family members. Don't take sides openly, even if you believe one person is right and the other is wrong.
  - Encourage the struggling parties to deal directly with one another.
  - Express your concern about each of them and your confidence that they can resolve their differences.
  - Don't fuel tensions between family members (or family members and friends, for that matter).
  - Don't sit in judgment on those who are at odds with one another.
  - If you're frustrated or angry with someone, deal directly with that person. Don't create a communication triangle by using someone else as your go-between.
  - Don't gossip about family members (or team members).
  - Be open and honest when you communicate with family and friends.

LOVE IS GOOD MEDICINE

Loving relationships may be the strongest ingredient in the prescription for living well with heart disease. If you are blessed with a close-knit family, celebrate one another often. If not, use the suggestions in this chapter to approach one another with newfound appreciation, and start treating one another with sensitivity and respect.

As for intimate partnerships: I cannot emphasize enough the critical importance of a happy primary relationship to your recovery. This is not just common sense; it's science. A Duke University study found that heart attack patients who were in long-term intimate partnerships had much lower death rates five years after the event compared to those who did not.[6] The companionship of someone who cares about you, someone in whom you can confide your deepest thoughts, fears, and hopes, will not only enrich your life but could actually save it.

If you try the strategies in this chapter but you and your family are still struggling, see a therapist. It's best if the family can attend together; if this isn't feasible, go with your partner, or go alone. Superb marriage and family counseling and marriage education (classes and workshops for married couples) are available throughout the country. You can ask your physician or rehabilitation specialist for a recommendation or contact the American Association for Marriage and Family Therapy, which can direct you toward qualified marriage and family therapists in your area (see Resources for contact information).

Chapter Five

EMBRACE YOUR NEW NORMAL
AND CULTIVATE
HEART-HEALTHY ATTITUDES

Recovering from heart disease requires that you make a decision to think differently than you did before—about life in general, your life in particular, and the attitudes you use to steer your way through it. This different way of thinking is an integral part of your new normal: rather than getting back to an old normal, you are moving *forward*, creating and embracing a new normal. You are redefining how you will approach and manage life from now on.

Why create a new normal? Because what was normal before a diagnosis of heart disease is often unhealthy and sometimes life-threatening afterward. A man known for his chronic crankiness before he developed heart problems could find himself dying from mismanaged anger later on. A pessimistic attitude is indirectly responsible for various kinds of health problems and seems to pose a direct threat to the heart.

In one study, scientists selected a group of 2,800 American adults and followed their medical ups and downs for more than twelve years. The results were sobering: those who reported feelings of depression or hopelessness were more likely to develop heart disease—both fatal and nonfatal—than those who weren't depressed.[1] Another study found that coronary bypass patients who were optimistic about the outcome of the surgery before the procedure returned to work sooner. Six months after the procedure, they reported a better quality of life in general than their less optimistic brethren.[2] The data led to an irrefutable conclusion: **If you want to recover from heart illness and thrive, you must adjust not only your physical habits but your psychological habits as well.**

Thriving with heart disease starts with this: you have to manage the way you think. You must examine and recast your thinking patterns because even remembering an upsetting event can have direct, negative effects on how well your heart works. Research has shown that when people with hardening of the arteries—arteries stiffened by deposits of fat, especially cholesterol—recall angry episodes, the hardened segments of their arteries constrict more severely (reducing the amount of blood they can accommodate) than the cleaner, more flexible segments.[3]

Martin Seligman is an expert on the health consequences of optimism, and his research along with others' has shown that health optimists don't only feel more cheerful, they also enjoy:[4]

- Better results from surgery
- Swifter recovery from surgery
- Improved mood, self-esteem, and overall happiness
- Happier and longer lives, regardless of their medical condition
- Less pain and fewer uncomfortable bodily symptoms
- Fewer infections

Optimists also tend to take better care of themselves in ways that promote cardiac health. For example, believing that what they do will indeed make a difference, optimistic heart patients are far more likely to go to the doctor, eat healthier foods, and exercise than are pessimistic patients, who see themselves as doomed to sickliness no matter what they do. They are also more likely to become information magnets and home in on news about their condition, such as the item that follows.

A NEW PREDICTOR OF HEART DISEASE: C-REACTIVE PROTEIN (CRP)

C-reactive protein, produced by the liver and within artery walls as a response to inflammation, has emerged as a predictor of heart disease that may be more reliable than elevated blood cholesterol levels. A landmark study published in *The New England Journal of Medicine* followed 28,000 women for an average of eight years and found that those with elevated CRP levels were more likely to suffer a first-time cardiovascular event such as heart attack or stroke than those with lower levels, even when their LDL, or "bad," cholesterol levels were low.[5]

We don't yet know whether CRP is a mere marker of cardiovascular risk or a cause. What we do know is that a simple blood test can tell you

---

if your CRP level is high enough to warrant concern, and your physician can tell you if your history and symptoms warrant having the test done. At this time, experts are not recommending that everyone be tested because the test now in use can give inconclusive results: a simple head cold can raise CRP levels, as can other harmless, noncardiovascular conditions such as a pulled muscle. And people who know they are likely candidates for heart illness probably won't learn anything new by having their CRP tested. But if you do have some risk factors (for instance, you weigh too much and your idea of exercise is power-walking to the refrigerator for a beer) and your cholesterol levels are normal, taking a CRP test could alert you to a risk you didn't know you had.[6]

If you're a negative thinker, you don't need the Oracle at Delphi to predict your future; negative thinkers fashion their own prophecies, which they fulfill with often fatal efficiency. If you sense pessimism in yourself, take note: if you don't do anything to improve your health, you are *greatly* increasing the odds that whatever risk factors you possess—including genetically linked health traits—will be magnified.

OPTIMISTS ARE MADE, NOT BORN

Are all well-adjusted heart patients natural-born optimists? Of course not. Some are, most aren't, but all of them work at cultivating positive, upbeat attitudes. Even heart patients who enjoy robust health sometimes indulge in negative thinking, which is often caused by stress. But they learn to catch themselves and replace pessimistic thought patterns with soothing, hopeful ones.

That's the great news: you *can* change the way you think; you *can* create new thinking patterns. You can conquer feelings of depression, anger, and hopelessness and go on to triumph over heart illness. Best of all, you can do it little by little: by making *small adjustments* to your attitudes, you can make *enormous* leaps toward full recovery.

One adjustment is to learn to recognize when you have slipped into a negative thinking rut and haul yourself out by thinking more positively, which usually means thinking more realistically. (If you're living in a negative thinking rut, you'll have a longer haul, but you can do it.) Start by paying attention to your thinking habits. Consider your thinking habits as you would other habits, such as biting your fingernails or saying "Um" too frequently. If you catch yourself biting your nails or saying "Um," you can learn to stop. Likewise, if you consciously catch yourself indulging in pessimistic thinking, you can learn to stop that, too.

Thinking pessimistically is like looking at the world through stress-colored glasses; the lenses distort your perceptions until your life reads like a worst-case scenario handbook. You distrust any stroke of good fortune, magnify trivial disappointments into conflicts, and turn challenging situations into calamities.

Here are descriptions of some typical negative thinking patterns that lead to the distortions I've just described. As you read, note any patterns that sound particularly familiar:

- **All-or-nothing thinking:** "I have a heart condition now, and I'll have a heart condition for the rest of my life. Nothing's going to change that."

- **Accentuating the bad, minimizing the good:** "Sure, I've quit smoking, but I've gained fourteen pounds and I don't fit into any of my jeans—not even my *fat* jeans. That's my life—one door closes, and another door closes."

- **Looking for something to worry about:** "Yes, my blood work looks good, and I am feeling stronger, but something is going to go wrong—I just know it. That's how my life is."

- **Mind reading:** "I've been living with you for seventeen years, and I know what you're thinking—you're sick and tired of me because I'm ill. I can tell."

- **If-I-feel-it-then-it-must-be-true thinking:** "I've been depressed since I came home from the hospital, and I've always been a cheerful person. If I feel this lousy, it must be because things are a lot worse than you're saying they are."

- **Blaming, shaming, and combinations of the two.**
  - **Blaming:** "This is all my fault. If I'd quit smoking when the doctor told me to, this never would have happened."
  - **Shaming:** "I'm not the only one responsible for this mess. Maybe if you'd quit smoking, I'd have been able to do it, too."
  - **Combination:** "I can't believe I brought this on our family. If we'd only tried harder to help each other quit, none of this would have happened."

If any of these examples hits home, look on the bright side: now that you've identified your negative thought patterns, you can start to change them. If none of them sounds quite like you, you're also in luck: you may have an easier time going through the following process of establishing your new normal thinking patterns.

The purpose of the process is to help you change negative patterns by taking three simple steps when your thinking veers toward the dark side:

1. Identify what you're feeling.
2. Identify the thoughts that are causing or complicating the feeling.
3. Look at the thoughts in a new, more realistic light (yes, that's your new normal).

You do this by asking yourself:

1. What am I feeling?
2. What thoughts are making me feel this way?
3. How can I look at these thoughts more realistically?

Let's say you've committed to eating healthier foods, summoned all your self-control, and haven't so much as looked at an onion ring or French fry in three months. You sail into the doctor's office and proudly await your blood work results—which reveal that your cholesterol level is still a bit too high. You sit there with your mouth in an *O,* figuring they must have mixed up your blood with someone else's . . . but no, it's your blood, and now it's starting to boil.

First, you ask yourself what you're feeling. Well, that's easy; you're angry as hell, confused, and more than a little worried. Next, you ask yourself what thoughts are making you feel that way, and your inner voice pipes up: *All that nonsense about eating healthier—it doesn't mean a thing. My cholesterol is still too high. I'm never going to get better!*

Finally, you view the thoughts in a new, more realistic light: *Okay. I'm not thrilled with my cholesterol count. But it's lower than last time, and at least we're tracking it now. I've got a good doctor, and he says I'm making fine progress. Maybe he's right. It took me a while to develop this problem, so it will take some time to fix it.*

HOW DO YOU FEEL ABOUT HAVING HEART DISEASE?

When you're creating new normal thought patterns, make sure you consider how you think about being a heart patient. It's very important that

MIND OVER MATTER? NOT ALWAYS

While your outlook on life does have a powerful effect on your health, remember that people do get sick for reasons that have nothing to do with their attitudes or psychological makeup. Even if we're lucky enough to live a long time, we all get sick and die. It's that simple.

Also remember that sometimes no amount of positive thinking will calm or comfort you. What you need most then is loving support—someone to listen to you, care about you, and hold you.

you give some thought to this, as your attitude toward the illness will influence how energetically you approach and conduct your recovery. Do you see the illness as a slap in the face or as a tap on the cheek that's awakened you to the importance of living more thoughtfully? Do you mark the diagnosis as an ending or a beginning? Do you feel as if you've been condemned to death or granted a second chance at life? (Hint: The hopeful choices are the healthy choices.)

WHAT IF A RECOVERY TEAM MEMBER HAS A NEGATIVE ATTITUDE?

It is profoundly discouraging for a recovering heart patient to be married to, live with, or be in close contact with a cynic. In these relationships, the optimistic person often squanders precious emotional energy neutralizing the cynic's disheartening remarks. But while a cynical team member may be hard to take, a proselytizing optimist is no picnic, either. If you're an optimist on a campaign to convert a downbeat team member, you risk dooming the very relationship you're trying to redeem.

A wiser approach is to accept one another's differences—to agree to disagree, if you will. Emotions are contagious, and families under stress are at increased risk of spreading negative emotions. Trying too hard to give a pep talk to a pessimist is likely to result in resentment and misunderstanding on both sides and deprive you of the support and comfort you both need.

This doesn't mean that you can't talk about your differences—which, by the way, won't be magically resolved by your united stand against the disease. Remember: intimacy does not imply sameness. Twin souls are not always the best soul mates; it's our differences that often bring us together and keep things interesting.

HOW DO THRIVING HEART PATIENTS THINK?

If you want to start thinking like a well-adjusted heart patient, here are some hints and reminders:

- **Consciously work at changing negative thought patterns to positive ones.** If ever there was a confirmed pessimist, it was Harold. When he was diagnosed with heart disease, he felt as if he'd just been given a death sentence. A fifty-eight-year-old accountant, Harold was accustomed to focusing on the bottom line, a habit he broke so he could start to mend his life:

"The first year after the diagnosis, I really struggled. I was bitter, angry, depressed. All I could think about were the things I wouldn't be able to do or eat or enjoy. If we went out to a restaurant, all I could think of was steak and that I wasn't allowed to order it. The truth is, steak was never my favorite thing, but now all I wanted was steak because I wasn't supposed to eat it.

"My wife finally gave me an ultimatum—either I got help or she'd get a divorce. So I got into group counseling—that was a shock. All these people telling me how cynical I am, pointing out how I'm always focusing on the negative aspects of an issue, never on the positive. I swear, until then, I'd never realized what a pessimist I was. I always thought I was naturally sarcastic, like I was born that way. The therapist running the group was good; she made me see how my cynical thinking was making me depressed, and not the other way around. And she showed me how to break my old habit of always seeing the negative aspects of things.

"It's pretty simple: I start out every day with five minutes of meditation—I relax, close my eyes, and picture my day going well. I imagine myself happy, handling situations smoothly, and I repeat to myself something like 'I have what it takes to make this a good day, even if things don't go the way I want them to. I have a lot to be grateful for—' and then I name four things I'm going to be consciously grateful for that day.

"It sounds corny, but it works. Reminding myself to think this way helps me calm down and notice the good stuff in my life—and there's a lot of it—and keeps me from obsessing about what's worrying me."

Cultivating an attitude of gratitude worked for Harold; other people achieve the same effect by repeating affirmations, gazing at photos of their grandchildren, meditating, or praying. There are as many methods as there are people. Do what works for you.

- **Reject New Age guilt.** The New Age movement has inspired a welcome wave of spiritual awareness but, along with it, some inaccurate, misguided, guilt-producing thinking. One popular myth is that if you're sick, it's because your parents didn't love you enough or because you actually *want* to be sick, since if you wanted to be well, you *would* be well.

  Thriving heart patients reject this lousy logic, and I urge you to reject it, too. You *do not* have heart disease because you unconsciously wanted to get it or because your spirit was too frail to repel it. *Why* you got it isn't as important as *how* you choose to live with it. Ditch any guilt in questioning why you're ill and harness your power to heal.

- **Don't blame yourself or others for the illness.** There's nothing to be gained from engaging in if-only thinking—if only I'd lost weight, if only you'd given up smoking, if only we'd tried harder. Don't look back in condemnation; look ahead with hope.

- **Accept that good is good enough.** Perfection is an unworthy goal because you'll never achieve it. Strive for adequacy—it's plenty good enough.

- **Keep things in perspective.** Don't inflate a quarrel into a catastrophe or disappointing blood work into a relapse. You don't need more drama in your life.

- **Catch yourself doing things right.** Focus on your successes, not your setbacks.

- **Work at maintaining an optimistic attitude.** Make a conscious effort to look for the good in every situation, every interaction, every moment. Your attitude affects numerous bodily conditions, including cholesterol level, blood count, immune function, the amount of acid your stomach secretes, and how much pain you feel. And positive expectations can affect how your body responds to medical treatments and procedures, including surgery.

CHANGING HEALTH BEHAVIORS FOR GOOD

Now you know how to think like a thriving heart patient; how can you change your habits to become one? You do it by recognizing the need to change, committing to making the change, making the change, and maintaining the change. This is the essence of creating and embracing a new normal.

I've devoted the rest of this chapter to introducing a four-step program that will give you the tools to start changing and keep you from getting overwhelmed. Briefly, the steps are:

1. Accept that changing is difficult and that you must develop your own way of doing it.

2. Understand that changing is a process, not a single decision or act.

3. Make changes in small increments (because little adjustments add up to big benefits).

4. Learn about and understand the stages of change.

Let's go over the program step by step.

1. Accept that changing is difficult and that you must develop your own way of doing it.

Everyone has his or her own style of changing a habit. Some begin to act in new ways and abandon old ones without obvious signs of struggle. These are the folks who crumple their cigarette packs, flush them down the toilet, and never light up again. Others jerk forward and backward in a series of starts and stops. They quit cold turkey, then start again, then cut back to half a pack a day, then use a nicotine patch, then taper off until they've stopped. Still others use the while-I'm-at-it strategy, which sounds something like this: "Quitting smoking will be tough. *While I'm at it*, I might as well start exercising, because it will keep me from gaining too much weight. And then, *while I'm at it*, I'll cut down on red meat and high-fat desserts, because that will also keep weight off and get my cholesterol down." Some people seek therapy to help them change. But most people change on their own, without professional help.

Regardless of your style, the key to creating lasting change in your life is believing that you have the ability to change. At the core of this belief is your confidence that your way of changing is a good one. This confidence is a necessity, because changing for good isn't easy. It takes work, and it takes time. Confidence breeds progress, and most people find that when they make progress in one area, they have more confidence to change in other areas.

2. Understand that changing is a process, not a single decision or act.

Changing a behavior isn't easy, and many factors go into making the new behavior stick. Of all the factors that can sabotage your attempts to change, the worst is that feeling of awkwardness you get when you're trying to replace an old habit with a new one. Many people mistakenly believe that in order for a change to be true and lasting, it must feel natural. The opposite is true. If you've ever tried to learn the proper way to swing a golf club, do the polka, use a computer, or conduct a civil discussion with your mate on a hot-button topic, you know that creating a new behavior pattern doesn't always feel natural, and sometimes it feels downright *un*natural.

To develop healthy habits that last a lifetime, you must live with the awkwardness until the change begins to feel real. Some of my patients like to use the "imagine it, act it, become it" technique, which loosely goes like this: if I can imagine an attitude, I can act as if I feel that way, and if I act that way long enough, I will become that way.

This technique instigates change from the outside in, and it works. Rather than requiring you to change your feelings first, the technique asks you to adjust your attitude and change your behavior, which is usually easier. The trick here is to be steadfast in the new behavior even in the early stages, when it isn't congruent with your feelings.

Three of my patients, Deborah, Selma, and Jake, talked to me about their experiences with this technique. Each of them was trying to change a different kind of behavior—Deborah, fifty-five, was trying to get more exercise; Selma, seventy-three, was trying to eat healthier foods; and Jake, sixty-one, was trying to become a better listener—yet they shared the same attitude: each of them felt like a fake.

"Who am I kidding?" Deborah asked. "I've never been athletic. What am I doing, acting like I'm a fitness nut?" Selma had a similar complaint: "Yes, I've lost eleven pounds, and yes, my cholesterol count has gone way down. But I still feel like a fat person who loves to eat junk food. How can this new me last when I feel as if I'm just faking it?"

Jake echoed the others: "I'm a pretty intense, hotheaded guy; always have been. Now I sit there, not saying a word, while Chris goes on and on and on, like I'm this perfect little listener. But I'm not—it's just not me. I feel like the biggest phony! How can Chris and I grow closer if I'm faking this listening stuff?"

Neither Deborah, Selma, nor Jake was faking. All three had decided they wanted to make the changes they were trying to grow accustomed to, and each was in the process of practicing a new behavior that didn't yet feel authentic. It is appropriate and necessary to go through a period when your new behaviors don't feel authentic; that's all part of creating a new normal. But if you practice long enough—typically for six to twelve months—new behaviors will lose their awkwardness and start to feel very normal indeed.

3. Make changes in small increments (because little adjustments add up to big benefits).

Here's more great news: you don't have to make grand, sweeping alterations to reap big benefits. You don't have to join an upscale health club or subsist on a diet of tofu and bean sprouts or enter a religious order to get fit, drop fat, and calm down. You can accomplish all these goals gradually, little by little, because small changes make you feel good, and good feelings inspire you to feel even better.

The strategy here is to start small and make minor modifications that, when linked in a growing chain, will connect you to your goal. For instance, if your goal is to quit smoking:

- Switch to a brand with lower tar and nicotine.
- If you smoke an unfiltered brand, start smoking one with a filter.
- Put out your cigarettes sooner.
- Calculate how many cigarettes you've cut out per day by putting out your cigarettes sooner.

If your goal is to get more exercise:

- Park your car farther and farther from the mall entrance.
- Take the stairs instead of the escalator once you get inside. At work, walk past the elevator and continue up the stairs (if you work on the twenty-seventh floor, start by walking up to the third floor and take the elevator from there; gradually work your way up more and more flights).
- Walk to the neighborhood bridge game instead of firing up the Thunderbird to go five blocks.

If your goal is to cut down on fats, lose weight, and eat more healthfully:

- Leave some of the high-fat food on your plate rather than finish it.
- Skip dessert, even if someone else is paying for the meal.
- Eat foods that are broiled; avoid those that are fried.

If your goal is to manage stress:

- When you complete a task, pause a few seconds or a even a minute or two before starting the next one.
- Let yourself sit in your car and finish listening to that song or program you're enjoying even if you've arrived at your destination.

- Take a night off—no work, no laundry, no paperwork, just recess.

If your goal is to increase your intimate connections with family members and friends:

- Before you launch into a recital of the ups and downs of your day, make a point of asking the person you live with how his or her day went—and *listen* when you get the answer.
- Throughout the day, carve out brief periods of time—say, thirty seconds each—of loving contact with someone you care about. Think of these as affection fiestas, if you will, in which you hug your kids and tell them you love them, tell a friend how great she looks and how much you appreciate her support, or look into your parents' eyes and let them know how much they mean to you.

4. Learn about and understand the stages of change.

No doubt you've heard the joke that goes "How many psychologists does it take to change a lightbulb? None—but the lightbulb really has to want to change." Well, it doesn't take a psychologist to change a heart patient, either; but the patient really has to want to change.

Your desire to change will empower you to change. You won't change until you're ready, no matter how much your partner, doctor, recovery team, and conscience beg you to. And once you're ready, you won't change all at once, magically arriving at your new behavior while the old one recedes in the distance. As you've seen, change is a process, not a done deal, and most people pass through a series of distinct stages on their way to making lasting changes in their lives. Your recovery will stay on track if you acquaint yourself with these stages and pay attention to your passage through them.

While there's no single paradigm that accommodates all patterns of change, psychologist James O. Prochaska has done a good job of identifying five phases that most people go through, which he calls the precontemplation, contemplation, preparation, action, and maintenance stages.[7] For our purposes, I've renamed the stages to show how heart patients typically respond when I ask them how ready they are to change a behavior pattern:

- **Stage I:** I don't need to change.
- **Stage II:** Sure, I'll change, but not right now.
- **Stage III:** I want to change, but I'm not sure how to start.

- **Stage IV:** Let's do it!
- **Stage V:** Now, if I can just keep at it.

Let's imagine someone who eats too much junk food and fast food, spends a lot of time in front of the TV, and needs to lose forty pounds. Here's how this person might progress through the stages of change.

STAGE I: I DON'T NEED TO CHANGE.

Everyone's telling me I've got to lose weight, but I don't want to.
If this sounds like you, you're not likely to change anytime soon. No matter how many people are nagging you, you won't lose the weight until you want to.

To move forward: Ask yourself why the people who care about you are encouraging you to lose weight. Then examine your reasons for saying you don't need to. Look at what you're likely to gain by dropping the weight versus what you're likely to lose by keeping it on. If you're honest, your reasons will seem very flimsy indeed and reveal themselves for what they are: excuses.

STAGE II: SURE, I'LL CHANGE, BUT NOT RIGHT NOW.

I know I should lose weight, but now is not the time.
If this sounds like you, you're making progress. You've consciously acknowledged that you need to change—a significant step toward creating change.

To move forward: Start learning about ways to make the change. Surrounding yourself with information (and the support of family and friends) will motivate you to press on. Here are some things you can do:

- Tell your doctor, therapist, or other medical professional that you want to lose forty pounds and ask for suggestions on how to start.
- Scour listings of community activities to learn about weight-loss lectures, clinics, and programs—and *go!*
- Join a support group such as Overeaters Anonymous.
- Visit a well-stocked newsstand and browse the shelves of colorful, upbeat magazines dedicated to teaching you to cook without fat and exercise without agony. (The major bookstore chains feature extensive magazine selections.)
- Read a book that addresses the issues involved in losing weight.
- Tell the members of your recovery team that you're thinking about embarking on a weight-loss program, and ask them to cheer you on.

Stage III: I WANT TO CHANGE, BUT I'M NOT SURE HOW TO START.

OK, I'm ready to get rid of the weight. How do I do it?

Once you're committed to making a change, you can start planning your strategy. In this stage, you prepare and motivate yourself for the ultimately liberating work ahead.

To move forward: Immerse yourself in an atmosphere charged with the possibility of change by looking at, listening to, and ingesting everything you can about what you plan to do.

- List the reasons why you want to change, emphasizing the benefits you will gain by changing. Post the list where you'll see it frequently, perhaps on the refrigerator door. For example, I want to start exercising regularly because doing so will:
  - Make my heart healthier
  - Help me feel more relaxed
  - Help me sleep better
  - Make me feel more attractive by toning my muscles daily
- Prepare to start by writing down exactly what you plan to do during the first week of your change program, noting **what** you will do, **where** you will do it, **when** you will do it, and **how long** you will do it. For example:
  - *What I'll do:* Walk Monday, Wednesday, Thursday, and Saturday next week.
  - *Where I'll do it:* At the Y's running track during the week, and in the neighborhood on Saturday.
  - *When I'll do it:* On my lunch hour during the week, and after breakfast on Saturday, before I run errands.
  - *How long I'll do it:* 30 minutes during the week, 45 minutes on Saturday.
- Review your plan and make sure the odds are good that you will follow through. Research shows that people follow through with an action *only when they are at least 70 percent confident they can do it.* In other words, if you think there's a fifty-fifty chance you'll have the gumption to stick to your plan, then chances are you won't. When this is the case, either modify your goal to make it more attainable or determine what would help you surmount the obstacles in your path.
- Promise yourself a reward for completing your plan. If you celebrate the small steps, you'll stay motivated throughout the journey.

CHANGE CONTRACT

I, _____, during the week of
_____, will do this activity or take this action:
_____
_____.

I will do it on the dates and at the times noted below:

Dates: _____,

Times: _____,

at the location(s) I have listed: _____
_____
_____.

My support person(s) will be _____
_____
_____.

I will reward myself for doing this by: _____
_____.

From 0 to 100 percent, I rate my confidence in my ability to complete this activity at:

[0% 10% 20% 30%] [40% 50% 60%] **[70% 80% 90% 100%]**

not   somewhat   very
confident   confident   confident

Adjust your contract until you are within the 70-100% very confident zone.

Here's how a completed one might look:

CHANGE CONTRACT

I, _____ *Morty Feinberg* _____, during the week of
_____ *September 15-21* _____, will do this activity or take this action:
Ride a bicycle, either mobile or stationary, four times for 35 minutes
each time .

I will do it on the dates and at the times noted below:

Dates: *Monday 9/15, Wednesday 9/17, Friday 9/19, and Sun. 9/21* ,

Times: *Mon., Wed., and Fri. at 7:30 a.m., and Sunday before noon* ,

at the location(s) I have listed: *Through the neighborhood, then up to Union*
Turnpike and back if the weather is good. If it isn't, I'll use the stationary
bike .

My support person(s) will be *Sarah—she's promised to ride with me on*
Sunday and maybe on other days too. If it's hot or rainy, she'll encourage me
to ride the stationary bike .

I will reward myself for doing this by: *Leaving work early one day next*
week and going to a Mets game .

From 0 to 100 percent, I rate my confidence in my ability to complete this
activity at:

[0% 10% 20% 30%]   [40% 50% 60%]   **[70% 80% 90% 100%]**

not   somewhat   very
confident   confident   confident

Adjust your contract until you are within the 70-100% very confident zone.

- Tell your recovery team that you're about to start your weight-loss program, and remind them to cheer you on.

STAGE IV: LET'S DO IT!

I can't wait to get this weight off!

Now that you're ready to change, make it easy on yourself. Don't be daunted by the enormity of the change you want to make; focus instead on small, manageable steps you can easily take. Remember, a journey of forty pounds begins with a single ounce.

To move forward:

- If your first-week goal is to exercise more, lay out your workout clothes the night before.

- Protect the time you've set aside to exercise. If a friend calls and wants to chat just as you're tying on your walking shoes, say, "Sorry, I can't talk right now. May I call you later?"

- If your goal is to cut out junk food, go through your cabinets and get rid of it.

- Commit to your new normal by signing a change contract with yourself. A few of my patients have balked at this, saying it feels too formal and that they'd prefer to make changes without writing it all down. I urge them to do it anyway, and I urge you to do it, too. Yes, it feels a bit unnatural, but that's part of creating a new normal, after all. Here are two copies of a change contract: a blank one, and one that's been completed by an imaginary New Yorker. Feel free to copy the blank one for your own use.

STAGE V: NOW, IF I CAN JUST KEEP AT IT.

I'm exercising regularly, eating better, and losing weight, but I still haven't lost my craving for fatty, junky foods. How do I make sure I don't fall back into my old ways?

Developing new habits takes time, and no one does it perfectly. Slipups and setbacks are part of the change process, not signs of failure. After all, statistics reveal that most reformed smokers tried to quit ten times before they quit for good. But they *do* manage to quit, and you, too, will manage to change deeply ingrained behaviors even if you suffer a setback now and then.

To move forward: Handle setbacks by seeing each one for what it is: a misstep, not a moral transgression.[8]

- Resist the urge to hate yourself for experiencing a setback and get back on track. Getting back on track boosts your confidence in your ability to stick with your change plan, no matter what it is you are trying to change.

- Minimize your vulnerability to setbacks by making your environment conducive to change. If you were trying to stop drinking, you wouldn't take a job in a liquor store. By the same token, if you're trying to stop eating junk food, don't keep your pantry full of cookies, chips, and candy bars.

  If you live alone, you can stock your pantry however you please. But if you live with a mate, let alone a kid or two, you can't purge your pantry of everything except wheat germ and rice cakes. This is where team support is so important. Explain to your family that you're trying to resist temptation and you need their help. Propose that the junk food items be stashed in a cabinet apart from the more healthy foods. If you don't have a cabinet to spare, remove the junk food from its original eye-catching packaging and disguise it in plain containers so it doesn't cry out to you every time you open the pantry door. And remember to thank the team for their cooperation.

- Identify situations that might shake your resolve before they occur, and prepare for them.

  Sam was a forty-eight-year-old divorced letter carrier whose heart attack shocked him into committing to an ambitious weight-loss program. But despite his enthusiastic attitude, his progress was inconsistent: after eating properly for several days, he'd slip back into bad habits for several more days before getting back on track. I asked Sam to focus on the upcoming week and identify situations that might threaten his resolve to eat properly. Here's what he came up with:

- Breaks at work
- Saturday-night dinners out
- Monday-night football

Then I asked Sam how confident he was he could stick to his plan in each situation. Sam said he felt 90 percent confident about work breaks and 80 percent confident about Saturday dinner, but only 30 or 40 percent confident about Monday-night football. Why? Because Sam's friends typically gathered at his house to watch the game on the big-screen TV, and Sam would stock up on snacks.

Sam decided that he needed to plan for these evenings long before his friends showed up. Here are the strategies he came up with:

- Don't have any junk food in the house.
- Have healthy snacks out during the game—a raw veggie platter prepared at the market; fresh fruit; popcorn, no salt or butter.

- Ask the guys to eat dinner before they come so we won't order pizza.
- Use setbacks to your advantage.

  - When you've suffered a setback, think back to the circumstances surrounding it and ask yourself: What is it about that situation (place, setting, relationship, conversation, dynamic) that puts me at risk of not following my plan?

  - When you've figured out what puts you at risk, prepare for the next time by telling yourself, "The next time I'm in that situation (place, setting, relationship, conversation, dynamic), it would help me stay on track if I could _____."

  Fill in the blank with a counterstrategy and *use it*.

- Beware of circumstances that commonly trigger setbacks. Negative emotions put you at risk of slipping back into undesirable habits. Anxiety, boredom, depression, or anger increases the odds that you will

  - Engage in an unhealthy behavior,
  - Sabotage a healthy behavior, or
  - Both.

  We are creatures of habit. If you have a twenty-year habit of lighting up a cigarette whenever you're on the phone, it's a good bet that every time the phone rings, you'll be reaching for your matches long after you've given up your Marlboros. So when the phone does ring, be prepared for that I'd-love-to-light-up feeling so it doesn't ambush you into searching your coat pockets for that old, broken half cigarette you meant to throw away (also, you might want to sign up for e-mail). And while I'm on the subject:

SMOKING KILLS HEART PATIENTS,
SO DON'T DO IT

Quitting smoking—not every few months, but *for good*—is the most forceful action you can take to save your life. Between 20 and 60 percent of heart attack survivors stop smoking, but only one-third to one-half of them stay stopped.[9] If you want a second opinion, go to *The New England Journal of Medicine:* a 1990 study published there indicated that heart attack survivors who continue to smoke are three and one-half times more likely to have another heart attack within the year than those who stop.[10]

ACCEPT THE FACTS (AND FLUSH YOUR PACKS)

If you smoke, be aware that:

1. Nicotine elevates your heart rate and blood pressure, and increases the likelihood that your heart will beat irregularly and that you will experience angina.
2. Nicotine increases blood clotting in your cardiovascular system.
3. A typical cigarette contains at least 43 different cancer-causing chemicals; when you light it, the number flares to 4,000.[11] These chemicals cause cancer and heart disease.
4. Carbon monoxide, one of the poisonous gases in cigarette smoke, damages the linings of your coronary blood vessels and increases the odds that you'll develop hardening of the arteries.
5. Both carbon monoxide and nicotine raise your levels of bad cholesterol and lower your levels of good cholesterol.
6. Within moments of taking a puff of a cigarette or a chew of tobacco, your heart rate increases by twenty-five beats per minute, both your systolic and diastolic blood pressure increase by twenty points, carbon monoxide chokes off oxygen in your blood, and nicotine shrinks the capacity of your arteries by half.

Don't be discouraged: others have quit smoking and you can, too. You know you must stop, and if you're like eight out of ten smokers, you've openly stated that you want to quit. In fact, you've probably quit several times already. **Most people try to quit ten times before they finally give up smoking for good.** And of the millions of Americans who have sworn off smoking, **90 percent did it on their own.**[12]

SOME FINAL HEARTFELT ADVICE

Start somewhere. Most heart patients start out feeling anxious and overwhelmed about all the changes they think they should make. You'll find the courage to start by picking something—*anything*—to change and starting there. Move forward every day, little by little. One day you'll look back and see how far you've come.

Chapter Six

LEARN TO MANAGE STRESS
AND IT WON'T HURT YOU

*(Because There's No Such Thing
as a Stress-Free Life)*

Roy and Carmine have several things in common. Both men are in their mid-fifties and suffered relatively mild heart attacks within the last three years. They work for the same textiles manufacturer, which recently was the object of an unusually hostile takeover. After the acquisition, both men were summoned for private meetings with their supervisors, who said how sorry they were to have to tell them their jobs were being eliminated. Roy and Carmine left the office that day with modest severance packages, a feeling of disbelief, and ninety days to find work.

While this wasn't good news for either Carmine or Roy, it was a lot worse for one man than the other. Because of their different ways of dealing with stress, one man would find himself wobbling on the brink of another heart attack, while the other man's heart would remain stalwart and strong.

ROY AND MARGO

To hear Roy tell it, the honeymoon was over before it began, when Margo squashed a slice of wedding cake into his face five minutes after promising she wouldn't. Margo rolls her eyes, weary of hearing this story yet again.

"You're such a victim," she says. "That was eighteen years ago! If it bothered you so much, why didn't you do it back to me?"

The couple is sitting in my office, stiff with tension and years of strife. They have come to see me at the suggestion of Roy's cardiologist, who thinks Roy's recent chest discomfort may be stress-related. It was Margo who called to make the appointment; she is the front office manager for a four-star hotel in town and has taken time off from work to be here.

Roy met Margo twenty years earlier, when he was thirty-five and she was twenty-eight. They had married swiftly and regretted it ever since. By the time I met them, their relationship had petrified into a stony edifice of mockery and rage grown even rockier since Roy's heart attack.

In an attempt to distract themselves from their differences, Roy and Margo had decided to build a new house. As they described the floor plan, I learned the house had five bedrooms, four bathrooms, a three-car garage, two fireplaces, and not a single thing they could agree on.

"What a fiasco," Roy says. "The framing is behind schedule, it's costing us fifty grand more than it's supposed to, and now I'm losing my job! I must have been out of my mind to think we could pull this off. Why are we even bothering?"

"Why are *we* bothering?" Margo says. "Dealing with this house is just like dealing with your illness; I'm doing all the work! You couldn't even be bothered to call the doctor. We wouldn't even be here if it weren't for me."

CARMINE AND BETTY

When you first meet Carmine and Betty, you're tempted to think in clichés: here's a happy, middle-aged couple with grown kids, a paid-off mortgage, and a weekly golf game. But they are anything but typical. Betty was a tenured professor of American Studies when she called Carmine's company to inquire about a fabric-dyeing technique she was researching. Carmine invited her to the plant and, according to him, it was "love at first sight— even though we both wore bifocals." Carmine was forty-six and a widower; Betty was forty-eight and, in her words, a contented academic. They married a year later and bought a house, but Betty kept her own place.

"We lived together in the home we bought," Betty says, "but I was nervous. I had a great little house—it was paid for, and I needed a safety net. I'd been living alone for over twenty years, and I didn't know if I could live with someone else."

Carmine was undaunted. "I figured she'd be fine, and she was. I gave her plenty of space. And for our first wedding anniversary, she gave me a great present—she put her house on the market, and it sold in a week."

But now Carmine says he wishes they still had that little house with the paid-off mortgage. The thought of having to live on a single income for a while is making them both anxious. Neither Carmine nor Betty was sleeping well, and they were both worried that Carmine would have another heart attack.

"I've got a couple of solid leads, but I've got to sound young on the phone so I can get an interview," Carmine says. "It's not easy for a geezer like me to get hired—"

"Here we go with the geezer routine," Betty says. "Listen—you're my trophy husband." And turning to me with a smile, "I love to show him off at faculty events."

Carmine takes Betty's hand and shakes his head. "Finally, at fifty-six, I'm a sex symbol," he says. "You know, it isn't easy. Two nights ago I lay awake all night, never fell asleep at all, but I was lucky—the next day was Sunday, so we went to church. And that's like another family; one person even got me an interview at her brother's company. I'm just so grateful for the support."

If you look at Roy and Carmine and compare the dynamics of their marriages and their resources for combating stress, you'll see exactly what I did: Roy is at far greater risk of suffering cardiac complications as a result of losing his job. He is caught in an ever-tightening vise: between building a house, battling with his wife, and looming unemployment, he is constantly at war with no furlough in sight. Carmine is more fortunate; although he is also losing his job, his heart is buffered by a battalion of defenders: a companionable marriage, a vibrant sense of humor, and the support of friends at church and elsewhere.

YOU *CAN* LEARN TO MANAGE STRESS, NO MATTER HOW STRESSED OUT YOU ARE

The great news is that, no matter how complex the causes of your stress may be, there are simple techniques you can use to protect yourself from the real danger—*strain* that evolves when you let stress go on too long.

About fifteen years ago, I recognized the futility of counseling patients to avoid stress. After all, who can live a life completely free of stress? Moreover, when you tell people to avoid something they start to fear it, and fear of stress causes a creeping psychological paralysis in heart patients that greatly increases their odds of experiencing another cardiac event or even early death. So instead of advising patients to avoid stress, I began alerting them to the actual causes of recurring cardiac events—psychological risk factors that I call the Big Five:

- Untreated depression
- Chronic anger or hostility (or both)

- Conflict with other people
- Social isolation
- Chronic anxiety

If you try to sidetrack stress by withdrawing from life, your psyche will stiffen into a breeding ground for these dangerous risk factors and multiply your odds of suffering additional cardiac events. That's the bad news.

The good news is that this doesn't have to happen: you *can* prevent long-term stress from eroding your health. And you accomplish this not by eliminating stress from your life—a scenario as undesirable as it is unrealistic—but *by taking manageable, concrete actions to control your stress reactions and prevent your stress from evolving into strain.*

I repeat: **Managing stress does not mean eliminating it but learning to control your reactions to it.**

WHAT IS STRESS?

Stress is what happens when you are confronted with the need to cope with a new situation. Stress is most apparent when there's a significant change in your life, bad or good. The stress of becoming a new parent can wrack your nerves as much as the death of your elderly mother or father, and a big promotion at work can be as vexing as learning you've been demoted. **The risk of a heart attack increases nearly tenfold for twenty-four hours after the occurrence of either an extremely desirable or an extremely undesirable event.**[1]

When stress hits, your mind and body react in ways that allow you either to deal immediately with what is stressing you or endure long-term stress reactions. Healthy stress—the sort that energizes and rejuvenates you—comes when you feel capable of mastering the challenge suddenly facing you. Put another way, healthy stress is characterized by a cultivation of the "three Cs": challenge, commitment, and control:[2]

- **Challenge:** You view change as invigorating, a new set of goals to strive for and achieve.
- **Commitment:** You commit yourself to meeting the challenge.
- **Control:** You equip yourself to exert control over yourself, your situation, and your recovery.

But unhealthy stress—the sort that overwhelms your sense of control and makes you feel incapable of coping effectively—can seriously damage your cardiovascular health. The question is, how much stress does it take to push you into the cardiac danger zone?

STRESS AND THE HEART:
SHORT-TERM RESPONSES AND RISKS

Living creatures—animals and humans alike—are born with an intricate network of nerves that regulates a vast array of bodily functions, including heart rate, breathing rate, blood pressure, and the expansion of large arteries that deliver oxygen-rich blood to the lungs. The sympathetic nervous system readies the body to respond to danger, and the parasympathetic nervous system calms everything down when the danger has passed.

When the sympathetic nervous system is activated, it triggers a host of bodily changes that we recognize as a stress reaction. Most of the body's immediate, short-term stress reactions are easy to detect and include pounding of the heart, tightness in the chest, sweating, headache, dry mouth, perspiring hands, and trembling muscles. You may also have an empty feeling in the pit of your stomach or feel nauseated; vomiting and diarrhea may also occur. These reactions happen when the body kicks into the fight-or-flight response:

- Stress hormones accelerate the heart rate, preparing you for action.
- Blood rushes toward the large muscles and away from internal organs so you can use your muscles to fight or flee.
- Blood vessels near the skin's surface constrict to minimize bleeding should you be wounded while fighting or fleeing.
- Muscles become tense, putting you on alert.
- The body becomes less sensitive to pain, preparing you for battle.

The short-term stress response was helpful long ago when fighting or fleeing predators was the only way to survive. Today, fight-or-flight is seldom an appropriate option when we feel threatened, yet our bodies are still hard-wired to respond this way. The result is that most people activate the stress response thirty to forty times each day without ever turning it off completely.

IS SHORT-TERM STRESS DANGEROUS TO YOUR HEALTH?

Yes and no. For more than twenty years, cardiologists have been debating whether or not a short burst of stress can cause a cardiac event. Some recent research indicates that it can:

- More than half of 224 heart attack patients admitted to a hospital said they had experienced stress or emotional upset shortly before admission.[3]

- You are five times as likely to suffer a heart attack after engaging in a strenuous exercise session as you were before the session, and your risk is even higher if you are unaccustomed to exercising.[4]

- An episode of intense anger more than doubles the risk that you'll have a heart attack during the next two hours.[5]

- In the month following the terrorist attacks of September 11, 2001, heart patients in the New York area suffered twice as many life-threatening heart-rhythm disturbances as they did in the month preceding the attack.[6]

Add to this the research revealing that any change in your activity level—including getting out of bed in the morning—increases your risk of having a heart attack,[7] and it's a wonder that any of us ever manages to change out of our pajamas.

But before you crawl back into bed, let's put these findings into perspective. First, bear in mind that although short bouts of stress do change the way the heart behaves, *most people who experience these stress-related changes do not develop heart illness.* After all, the vast majority of us do get out of bed, fold our pajamas, and leave the house. Further, even though exercising moderately may raise your risk of heart attack for an hour after the session, exercising regularly *dramatically reduces* your risk of heart attack for the 167 remaining hours of the week.

Perhaps most important is the reassurance offered by psychologist Robert Allan and cardiologist Stephen Scheidt, who assert that the odds that a fifty-year-old man with no coronary risk factors will have a heart attack in any given hour is approximately *one in a million*—very low odds.

But what about the stress statistics I cited a few minutes ago? Well, let's imagine that our fifty-year-old friend is driving home in rush-hour traffic in his '96 sedan, gets cut off by a late-model sports car, and experiences, shall we say, an episode of anger. According to Drs. Allan and Scheidt, the odds of him having a heart attack would go up to only *2.3 in a million*—still very low odds.[8] The implication is clear: a single stress response is rarely dangerous to the health of your heart; if you become stressed and then calm down, there is usually no damage.

But what if you don't calm down? What if a typical day finds you tensing up in a series of stressful encounters and the parasympathetic nervous system never has a chance to properly calm you? And what if this goes on for days, weeks, months, or even years?

That's when you run into trouble.

STRESS AND THE HEART:
LONG-TERM RESPONSES AND RISKS

When the stress response is activated again and again and you don't turn it off between episodes, you enter the cardiac danger zone, where your long-term stress pattern drives you into higher and higher levels of *strain*. Strain develops when daily hassles outnumber uplifts. We now know that minor irritants that accumulate over time threaten health more than the occasional major life event.[9] And research has shown that enjoying small pleasures frequently will do more to improve your mood than sporadic bursts of elation.[10] So even when you're experiencing a great deal of negative stress, you can safeguard your health and happiness by making sure each day contains at least one oasis of pleasure, however simple.[11]

Living with strain over time can hurt you in many ways:

- We've known for some time that unchecked strain can render the body's immune system more vulnerable to infections and illnesses such as cancer. But new research goes further and suggests that disturbing the immune system may also cause inflammation that contributes to the development of coronary artery diseases.[12]

- If the hormones that flow during a stress response are repeatedly pumped into your body, they can raise blood levels of LDL (bad cholesterol) and lower levels of HDL (good cholesterol). Stress hormones also increase the odds that artery wall linings will accumulate clots that harden into atherosclerotic plaque, a condition called atherosclerosis, or hardening of the arteries.

- When you're under stress for a long time, the brain centers that control physical reactions—for example, the hypothalamus—cause your blood pressure to gradually rise.[13]

- As long-term stress becomes strain and alters the functioning of the nervous system, the risks of heart attack, ischemia, or sudden death increase. (Ischemia occurs when the heart muscle does not receive enough oxygenated blood to fuel its pumping. About half of cardiac patients experience episodes of ischemia associated with mental stress.)[14]

- Chronic worriers who also have high levels of anxiety are more likely to suffer from elevated blood pressure, increased risk of arrhythmia (unstable heart rhythm) and sudden death from a heart attack. In fact, chronically anxious people are two to four times more likely to die from a cardiac event than those who are able to calm their stress reactions.[15]

- Chronic stress also impairs the heart's ability to pump blood to the lungs for oxygen and then propel the oxygenated blood throughout the body.[16]

Once again, the implication is clear: living with stress for a long time can lead to heart disease and it **may lead you to a premature death once you have it.** Moreover, as with physical risk factors, **the more psychological risk factors you combine, the more likely it is that stress will cause you to have a cardiac event.** Psychiatrist Redford Williams of Duke University Medical Center and historian Virginia Williams are experts in the field of anger research and have noted that several risk factors, each of which is dangerous to heart health in and of itself, tend to gather in certain individuals:

- Hostility, depression, and social isolation
- Repeated activation of the stress response
- Lack of calming after activation of the stress response
- Poor health habits and behaviors [17]

Note that all these risk factors are well within your ability to change and control—something we'll get to shortly. But first I want to talk about two other factors that are so obvious they are often overlooked: toxic work environments and vital exhaustion.

IS YOUR JOB TOXIC?

From time to time, we all criticize our jobs for being frustrating, challenging, difficult, boring, demanding, ridiculous, and paying way too little—and from time to time, we're all correct. But it turns out that some jobs can actually be toxic to your heart, and you should take a few minutes to figure out if yours is one of them.

In a now-classic study, a team of scientists spent six years tracking the health patterns of nearly two thousand working Swedish men and radically changed our way of thinking about work and stress. Their results showed that the men who were most likely to develop heart disease were those whose jobs were highly demanding but which allowed them little control over either the pace or outcome of the work.[18] Since then, researchers have shown that high-demand/low-control stress is also implicated in raising blood pressure as well as death rates from various causes, not just heart illness. These findings are chilling, considering how many people feel they have little control over what their jobs require them to do, or how they are permitted to do it.

Take a few minutes now to evaluate the stress risks of your job by completing the following questionnaire, which is adapted from one used by the Swedes. And if you're a homemaker, this questionnaire is for you, too—you certainly have a job, even if you don't get sick days (and please don't laugh too hard when you get to question K).

KARASEK JOB STRAIN QUESTIONNAIRE[19]

Use the following scale to answer each question as it applies to your job:

Strongly disagree   1

Disagree   2

Agree   3

Strongly agree   4

A. My job requires that I learn new things.   ____

B. My job requires a high level of skill.   ____

C. My job requires that I be creative.   ____

D. My job requires that I do things over and over.   ____

E. I have freedom to decide what I do on the job.   ____

F. I decide how much of the job gets done.   ____

G. My job requires that I work fast.   ____

H. My job requires that I work very hard.   ____

I. I am not required to complete excessive amounts of work.   ____

J. I have enough time to get the job done.   ____

K. I am free of requests that place conflicting demands on my time.   ____

Total: ____

SCORING THE KARASEK JOB STRAIN QUESTIONNAIRE

This is one of the more complex scoring systems you'll ever see, but it is interesting. Even so, feel free to complete the questionnaire and skip the scoring. I'll help you interpret your results either way.

1. Add your scores in questions A, B, and C:

    ____ (A) + ____ (B) + ____ (C)   = ____

2. Subtract your score in question D from five (5): 5 − ____ (D) = ____

3. Add the results of steps 1 and 2, above: (step 1) + (step 2)   = ____

4. Add your scores in questions E and F, and multiply the sum by two (2):

    ____ (E) + ____ (F) = ____ × 2   = ____

5. Add the results of steps 3 and 4 to arrive at Subtotal I:

    ____ (step 3) + ____ (step 4) Subtotal I   = ____

6. Add your scores in questions G and H: ____ (G) + ____ (H) = ____

7. Multiply the result of step 6 by three (3) to arrive at Subtotal II:

    ____ (step 6) × 3 Subtotal II   = ____

8. Add your scores in questions I, J, and K:

    ____ (I) + ____ (J) + ____ (K)   = ____

9. Subtract the result of step 8 above from fifteen (15):

    15 − ____ (step 8)   = ____

10. Multiply the result of step 9 above by two (2):

    ____ (step 9) × 2   = ____

11. Add up the results of step 7 (Subtotal II) and step 10 above

_____ (Subtotal II)

+ _____ (step 10)

Grand total: _____

INTERPRETING THE QUESTIONNAIRE

Subtotal I quantifies how much decision latitude you feel you have in your job. Decision latitude refers to how much freedom you have to make decisions and determine your schedule, meaning both the hours you're expected to be at work and the way you spend your time when you're there. Scores can range from 8 (low decision latitude) to 32 (high decision latitude). A score lower than 24 means you feel you have little control over how you perform your job.

The grand total refers to how psychologically demanding you think your job is. Scores for this section range from 12 to 48, with a score of 32 or higher indicating that you find your job to be psychologically demanding.

Is it stressful to have a psychologically demanding job? Not necessarily. The amount of stress you feel depends on how much decision latitude or control you have. When you score the questionnaire, look at the relationship between the two scores—that's the key to analyzing your job strain quotient. If you feel you have low decision latitude but your job isn't psychologically demanding, your job stress level may be comfortably low. If your job requires rigorous mental activity but affords you high decision latitude, your stress level may also be low. But if your job imposes psychological burdens without empowering you to make decisions, your job may be a source of strain.

Even if you choose not to score the questionnaire, just reading it makes the point that many factors combine to create high-demand/low-control work stress. Also remember that many factors not mentioned in the questionnaire can contribute to work stress, including low job security, inadequate pay, conflicts with coworkers, clients, or customers, irregular and unpredictable schedules, and the difficulties of juggling family and work demands.

Finally, remember that high-demand/low-control stress is not limited to toxic work settings. If you feel that any important aspect of your life is out of control, you're bound to feel the strain.

VITAL EXHAUSTION

For years I've heard heart patients say that when they look back, they realize there were clues that they were going to have a heart attack or other cardiac event. In addition to familiar symptoms such as chest pain and shortness of breath, they also reported feelings of fatigue and general discomfort, a condition we have come to know as *vital exhaustion*. You may be suffering from vital exhaustion if

- You feel unusually fatigued.
- Your energy level has gone down.
- You feel exhausted when you wake up in the morning.
- You feel dejected or defeated much or all of the time.
- You're more easily irritated than usual.
- Your sex drive has abated or disappeared.

Vital exhaustion is not the same as depression, although some symptoms of depression, such as loss of energy and sex drive, may be associated with it. The key difference is that people with vital exhaustion do not typically suffer from feelings of guilt or lowered self-esteem.[20] Nor is it the same as fatigue, as you cannot banish vital exhaustion by getting a good night's sleep, but must change the behavior patterns that drained your energies in the first place.

Vital exhaustion is now regarded as a reliable predictor of heart illness because of the Dutch study that identified the syndrome. Researchers followed nearly four thousand employees of the city of Rotterdam over four years and found that those who manifested symptoms of vital exhaustion were more than twice as likely to have a heart attack as those who did not.[21]

A more recent study followed patients who underwent coronary angioplasty to repair a damaged blood vessel. (In angioplasty, a tube with a tiny balloon at the tip is threaded into an artery blocked by a buildup of plaque. The balloon is then inflated at high pressure to flatten the obstruction; after a minute or so, the balloon is deflated, the tube removed and, if all has gone well, the artery is clear.) A year and a half after angioplasty, fifteen of forty-three vitally exhausted patients had suffered a new cardiac event, compared to fourteen of eighty-four nonexhausted patients—in other words, the patients suffering from vital exhaustion were twice as likely to suffer another cardiac event as were the more robust patients.[22]

ARE YOU SUFFERING FROM VITAL EXHAUSTION?

I have printed below an adaptation of the Maastricht Questionnaire, named for the Dutch study in which it was used. Completing the questionnaire will give you an idea of whether or not you are suffering from vital exhaustion.

The questionnaire consists of questions that ask you to think about how you have been feeling lately. Answer each question as best you can, circling "Y" for yes and "N" for no; if you're not sure about an answer, circle the question mark. Please note that there is no clear-cut formula for tabulating the answers to this instrument; nor are there any right or wrong answers.

THE MAASTRICHT QUESTIONNAIRE [23]

1. Do you often feel tired?	Y	N	?
2. Do you frequently have trouble falling asleep?	Y	N	?
3. Do you wake up repeatedly during the night?	Y	N	?
4. Do you feel weak all over?	Y	N	?
5. Do you feel you haven't accomplished much lately?	Y	N	?
6. Do you feel you can't cope with everyday problems as well as you used to?	Y	N	?
7. Do you believe you have come to a dead end in life?	Y	N	?
8. Do you feel more listless than you used to?	Y	N	?
9. Do you enjoy sex less than you used to?	Y	N	?
10. Do you feel hopeless and demoralized?	Y	N	?
11. Does it take you longer to grasp a difficult problem than it did a year ago?	Y	N	?
12. Do little things irritate you more than they used to?	Y	N	?
13. Do you feel like giving up?	Y	N	?

14. If someone asked how you were feeling, could you
honestly say, "I feel fine"?   Y   N   ?

15. Does your body sometimes feel like a battery that's
losing its power?   Y   N   ?

16. Do you sometimes wish you were dead?   Y   N   ?

17. Do you feel you no longer have what it takes?   Y   N   ?

18. Do you sometimes feel like crying?   Y   N   ?

19. Do you ever awaken in the morning feeling exhausted? Y   N   ?

20. Is it increasingly difficult for you to concentrate on
a single subject for a long time?   Y   N   ?

As I mentioned, this questionnaire doesn't come with a scoring formula. Rather, its authors designed it to stimulate people to think about feelings and complaints that could signal the advent of vital exhaustion.

As you read the questionnaire, you may notice that many of the symptoms describe conditions common to people who are depressed, cynical, or hostile. Indeed, these factors have been found to increase the risk of developing or dying from coronary heart disease. But the syndrome of vital exhaustion is an especially astute predictor of heart illness—far more than depression, cynicism, or hostility.

Finally, remember that *merely being in a state of vital exhaustion will not cause you to have a heart attack or any other cardiac event.* It's when you combine vital exhaustion with other risk factors that you enter the stress danger zone.

FOUR STEPS TO MANAGING STRESS

As I said earlier, you can use simple strategies to alleviate long-term stress and strain and preserve your health. The rest of this chapter will acquaint you with my four-step program for managing stress, which asks you to:

1. Identify your stress reactions.

2. Make small changes in your stress reactions.

3. Avoid five classic stress-boosting behaviors.

4. Massage your mental muscles with stress-shrinking techniques and activities.

Let's go over the steps one by one.

1. Identify Your Stress Reactions.

Many people confuse stress with anxiety. They figure if they're not nervous and jittery, they must not be stressed. Right?

Not necessarily. Stress affects different people in different ways, and the first step in the program is to identify how stress affects you. To do this, I have included a series of forms that ask you to note your physical, mental, emotional, behavioral, and interpersonal reactions to stress. Let's get started.

Bring to mind an event that you recall as stressful—a situation of importance that confronted you with change, whether pleasant or unpleasant—and ask yourself:

a. What did my body feel like? (Identify your physical stress reactions.)

b. What feelings did I have? (Identify your emotional stress reactions.)

c. How was I thinking? (Identify how your thinking reacts to stress.)

d. How did I act? (Identify how your personal behaviors react to stress.)

e. How did I interact with others? (Identify how your interpersonal behaviors react to stress.)

a. *What did my body feel like? (Identify your physical stress reactions.)*

In response to the stressful event, I experienced:

___ Rapid heartbeat	___ Shallow breathing
___ Tense shoulders or back	___ Twitching muscles
___ Heartburn	___ Bowel problems
___ Dry mouth	___ Jaw pain
___ Headaches	___ Backaches
___ Skin problems	___ Hives
___ Insomnia	___ Excessive fatigue
___ Elevated blood pressure	___ Tearing eyes
___ Excessive perspiration	___ Feeling flushed

___ Excessive appetite   ___ Loss of appetite
___ Dizziness   ___ More intense focus
___ Other _____
___ Other _____

b. *What feelings did I have? (Identify your emotional stress reactions.)*

In response to the stressful event, I felt:

___ Sad   ___ Lonely   ___ Angry
___ Anxious   ___ Disgusted   ___ Contemptuous
___ Manic   ___ Energized   ___ Fearful
___ Discouraged   ___ Helpless   ___ Shy
___ Paralyzed   ___ Scattered   ___ Numb
___ Other _____
___ Other _____

c. *How was I thinking? (Identify how your thinking reacts to stress.)*

In response to the stressful event, my thinking featured the following characteristics:

___ Worrying   ___ Worst-case-scenario thinking
___ Blaming myself   ___ All-or-nothing thinking
___ Blaming others   ___ Negative or cynical thinking
___ Obsessive thinking   ___ Difficulty concentrating
___ Angry thoughts   ___ Self-pitying thoughts
___ Thinking like a victim
___ Other _____
___ Other _____

d. *How did I act? (Identify how your personal behaviors react to stress.)*

In response to the stressful event, my personal behaviors featured the following characteristics:

___ Rushing   ___ Slowing down
___ Eating too much   ___ Eating too little
___ Sleeping too much   ___ Sleeping too little

___ Working too much   ___ Working too little

___ Smoking   ___ Drinking too much alcohol

___ Driving aggressively   ___ Using illegal substances

___ Exercising compulsively   ___ Growing sedentary

___ Running from reality   ___ Procrastinating

___ Other _____

___ Other _____

e. How did I interact with others? (Identify how your interpersonal behaviors react to stress.)

In response to the stressful event, when interacting with others I tended to behave in the following ways:

___ Argumentative   ___ Aggressive   ___ Overly affectionate

___ Defensive   ___ Controlling   ___ Passive

___ Uncooperative   ___ Sarcastic   ___ Competitive

___ Overly sensitive   ___ Overeager   ___ Needy

___ More assertive   ___ Bored   ___ Brusque

___ Unaffectionate   ___ Less assertive   ___ Hurried

___ Other _____

___ Other _____

Now I want you to summarize in a few sentences what you learned about each of your stress reactions. For instance, if you checked off *argumentative, sarcastic, aggressive, brusque,* and *defensive* in Section e, as ways you interact with others when you're under stress, you might write: "When I'm stressed, I act as if I'm angry with people, like I want to pick a fight. It's a way of keeping everyone at a distance."

Fill out each section, using more paper if you need to.

a. *Summary: How my body reacts to stress*

Which of your body systems reacts most strongly to stress and strain? Where do you take stress hits?

_____

_____

_____

_____

_____

b. *Summary: How my emotions react to stress*
How do you feel when you are stressed?

_____
_____
_____
_____
_____

c. *Summary: How I tend to think when I am stressed*

How does stress affect the way you think?

_____
_____
_____
_____

d. *Summary: How I act when I am stressed*

How does stress affect the way you act?

_____
_____
_____
_____

e. *Summary: How I treat others when I am stressed*

How does stress affect the way you interact with others?

_____
_____
_____
_____

If you had trouble writing these summaries, observe yourself for several weeks, noticing how your body, emotions, thoughts, and behaviors react to stress and indicate when it's building up. Picture these reactions as dominoes standing on edge and close to one another in a long, snaking row. And remember that all it takes is one domino—one risk factor too many—to tip the next one over, and the next tips the next, until the row of dominoes collapses, one by one. But—as always—I have good news: when you change one of your stress reactions, you move that domino just a little farther away from its neighbors, so even if it tips over, it's less likely to tip the next one. By managing your reactions, you protect your heart from collapsing under the strain of long-term stress.

2. Make Small Changes in Your Stress Reactions.

In the last chapter, I said that small steps add up to big benefits, and the same is true for stress: making small changes in your stress reactions will make a big difference in breaking the stress-strain progression. The happiest and healthiest people aren't blessed with extraordinarily good fortune, but they do devote more energy to basking in life's pleasures than they do to clenching their teeth over its letdowns. You too can manage stress by:

- Cultivating a positive attitude
- Countering your stress reactions with the relaxation response
- Treating yourself to simple, healthy pleasures

The Relaxation Response

Both the stress response and the relaxation response are natural body reactions: the stress response readies you for action, and the relaxation response enables you to recover. But whereas the stress response turns on automatically, you must deliberately trigger the relaxation response. And there are many ways to trigger it: exercise, diaphragmatic breathing, meditation, yoga, visualizing yourself in a tranquil setting, getting a massage, enjoying sexual relations, recalling a calming experience, and praying can all relax you.

Relaxation is good for you: it lowers your heart rate and breathing rate, enhances concentration, eases muscle tension, allows you to sleep more deeply, lowers your awareness of pain, calms anxiety, and boosts the functioning of your immune system. It also lowers your risk of developing heart disease, and bolsters your ability to recover from it.

One of the best ways to trigger the relaxation response is through diaphragmatic, or stomach breathing. I recommend you learn this technique not only because it works, but because you can use it anytime, anywhere, without anyone knowing.

Diaphragmatic Breathing

The diaphragm is a large, dome-shaped muscle in the abdomen. When you breathe from the diaphragm, you inhale into your belly and expand this muscle, which is how newborn babies breathe (and how we would all still breathe were we not taught to push out our chests like good little soldiers). To find your diaphragm, place your palm on your abdomen, just beneath the rib cage. Then inhale, pushing your hand out—that's your diaphragm. If you're not sure you're doing it correctly, place your other hand on your chest when you inhale. When you're breathing from the diaphragm, the hand on your chest will remain still, and the hand on your abdomen will push out.

Some people find it easier to locate the diaphragm by lying flat on the floor, placing a book on the abdomen, and making the book rise as they inhale. It seems counterintuitive at first, but keep at it until you are able to inhale while expanding your belly. When the book rises, you're breathing from the diaphragm.

What's so good about diaphragmatic breathing is that you're taking in more air than you can when you breathe into your chest, so you don't have to inhale as frequently to get the oxygen you need. As a result, your breathing rate slows, your heart rate slows, and you relax. Moreover, it's an invisible technique— you can do it while sitting at dinner or at a meeting, while you're waiting in line at the market, at your grandchild's softball game, or while you're conversing with a dinner companion. You're also taking deliberate action to control your body, a fundamental part of thriving with any illness.

Breathing from the diaphragm is the natural way to breathe, but most of us have to relearn it after years of breathing differently, and it takes time. Be patient with yourself and allow three or four weeks to master this technique. Remember that you're learning a new habit while unlearning an ancient one—chest breathing—that you've been practicing for decades.

Muscle Relaxation

Another way to trigger the relaxation response is to relax your body by systematically tensing and releasing each muscle group. While not as subtle as diaphragmatic breathing, this technique is particularly effective when used in conjunction with it, and you can practice a toned-down version without anyone noticing you're doing it.

To begin, sit in a comfortable chair with your feet on the floor or lie down (yes, the technique is more noticeable if you lie down). If you're sitting, let your arms and hands rest in your lap; if lying down, let your arms rest at your sides. Take several deep, cleansing breaths. Then inhale and, starting with your feet, tense each muscle group, hold it tightly for five seconds, and then release. Move up from your feet to your calves, thighs, buttocks, abdomen, hands, forearms, upper arms, shoulders, neck, and face (don't do your face muscles if you're in public and don't want people to notice). Isolate each muscle group as best you can, tense it independently of the others, hold it, and exhale when you release. Take two or three deep breaths between each group.

Simple, Healthy Pleasures

Muscle relaxation and diaphragmatic breathing are two calming techniques; there are many others. Some people quiet themselves by engaging in meditative activities such as knitting, painting, or gardening. Others close their eyes and guide themselves on an inner journey, visualizing a pleasant time, place, or event that invokes serenity. Heart health and the experience of pleasure are tightly linked, and a crucial component of your recovery is your willingness to allow yourself to feel pleasure.

It's a necessity, not a luxury—at least according to psychologist Robert Ornstein and physician David Sobel, who claim that enjoying simple, healthy pleasures is the key not only to better stress management but to better overall health.[24] Most people don't realize that

- A hug or a massage can lower your heart rate.
- Taking a hot bath or sauna lowers stress hormones and blocks pain.
- Spending time in sunshine can improve your mood (but not your skin—do apply sun-block).
- Viewing nature can relax you.
- Pleasing sounds such as those found in nature and soothing music lower anxiety and pain.
- Agreeable scents can elevate your mood (as evidenced by the popularity of aromatherapy).
- Regular exercise helps your body defuse stress reactions and turn on the relaxation response more quickly.
- As simple an activity as a walk around the block can ease tension.
- Using less caffeine and alcohol can lower your levels of anxiety, tension, and strain.

This last item brings us to the third step in the stress reduction plan: resisting choices and actions that heighten stress.

3. AVOID FIVE CLASSIC STRESS-BOOSTING BEHAVIORS.

I have known many heart patients who sabotaged their recovery plans by succumbing to stress-boosting behaviors. Here are the five I see most often, which I advise you to avoid:

1. **Don't run from your problems (do face them).** Take breaks from worry and work to manage your stress, but pay attention to what kinds of breaks you take.

    - **Avoid escapes into oblivion.** Numbing your stress with drugs, alcohol, nicotine, or food will weaken your resolve, make you dependent, and increase, not diminish, your stress.

    - **Don't go numb—have the courage to feel.** If you ignore fatigue, worry, fear, anxiety, sadness, grief, and other emotions, you distance yourself from bodily and psychological sensations and diminish your awareness of both what's happening to you and what you must do to feel better.

2. **Don't speed up (slow down instead).** When we're under pressure, we tend to speed up rather than slow down—exactly the opposite of what we should do. Increasing your speed only ratchets up your stress. Make yourself pause and breathe deeply—even if it's just for a minute—and *relax* before continuing your activity.

3. **Don't wait until . . . (do act now).** I seldom meet a heart patient who doesn't regret waiting too long before taking better care of him- or herself. The wait-until syndrome comes in many flavors, some of which you may have tasted:

    - "I'll wait until the new year; then I'll start taking better care of myself."

    - "I'll wait until I lose some weight; then I'll feel attractive enough to join the health club."

    - "I'll wait until I feel better; then I'll start to enjoy my life." (If you wait, you may not get the chance.)

4. **Don't give up (do persevere).** My patients sometimes complain, "As soon as I calm down about one thing, another comes up. What's the use of trying to ease my stress when it just keeps coming?" Stress will keep coming your way, but remember your goal is not to eliminate stress but to change the way you react to it. That is something you can control, and you owe it to yourself not to give up.

5. **Don't become chained to one coping strategy (do adapt your strategy**

to the situation). Two kinds of coping strategies, taking action (problem-focused coping), and self-soothing (emotion-focused coping), will help you manage stress if you match the strategy to the situation. If you don't, you'll make things worse. The trick, of course, lies in knowing which one to use.

Taking action is helpful when the stress-causing problem is something you can remedy yourself, something within your power to control. For example, if you're stressed because your house is messy, the problem (messy house) can be remedied by taking action (tidying up). Or if you're anxious that you might suffer another cardiac event and want to minimize your risks, you can take action by exercising regularly and improving your eating habits.

But what if the problem is *not* something that is under your control? What if you're worried because your daughter is determined to marry someone whose considerable character flaws are obvious to you but not to her? Or your brother's emphysema is worsening while he still smokes a pack of cigarettes a day and warns you not to mention it? Or if you're wracked with anxiety because you're facing another surgery and hospital stay to repair a faulty heart valve?

There is no action you can take to eliminate these sources of stress, so a problem-focused coping strategy won't work: you can't stop your loved ones from doing things that worry you. The next best thing is to *put your energy into soothing your reactions to the stress rather than struggling to change the situation that is causing it.* Adjust your strategy: instead of focusing on the problem and leaping into potentially harmful action, focus on the emotion (your worry, anxiety, and stress) and use one or more of these self-soothing techniques:

- Reassure yourself that you're doing all you can to deal with the problem.

- Distract yourself from your discomfort by indulging in healthy pleasures.

- Get support and encouragement from friends and relatives.

- Use relaxation techniques, prayer, meditation, or whatever works for you to calm down and keep things in perspective.

- Reframe the problem. In other words, view the issue in a way that calms your anxieties. For example, instead of seeing your daughter's upcoming marriage as the event that will ruin her life unless you can stop her, see it instead as *her* necessary journey, one you cannot—and should not—protect her from.

This is not a precise science; no strategy is unconditionally guaranteed to soothe stress reactions. But by adapting your strategy to the stress, you won't make matters worse, and you might make them better.

4. MASSAGE YOUR MENTAL MUSCLES WITH STRESS-SHRINKING TECHNIQUES AND ACTIVITIES.

The fourth step of my stress management plan asks you to calm yourself consciously by participating in everyday activities and techniques that shrink stress. Here is a list of my top choices; you've already heard about some of them, but they're worth repeating:

1. **Manage your attitude.** Pay attention to how you interpret daily events, examine your reactions to others, and don't flinch from your less-than-sunny moments. Being hopeful is a choice; choose hope.
2. **Lower your general stress level.** The most obvious way to stay out of the strain zone is to keep your stress level low enough that even a stress spike won't kick you there.
3. **Cultivate your sense of humor.** A good laugh lowers stress hormones, relaxes you, and helps you keep problems in perspective.
4. **Try to maintain balance among the major orbits of your life:** work, family, community, self. That said, take heed of point number 5.
5. **Reject the myth of the perfectly balanced life.** Don't get taken in by those stories you read about people whose exquisite skill enables them to painlessly juggle romance, marriage, children, and career while caring for their ailing in-laws, volunteering at the local soup kitchen, earning a college degree at night, and fulfilling everyone else's needs. Healthy people enjoy working hard at what they love, and this sometimes takes them away from the people they love. *Perfect balance is neither possible nor necessary.* Every life is a little lopsided. The key: don't ignore any area of your life for too long.
6. **Treat yourself to simple, healthy pleasures.** You've read about what these are. Indulge yourself in them.
7. **Take frequent mini–relaxation breaks throughout the day.** Whether you're at work, at home, or out and about: before moving on to your next task, pause for a minute, close your eyes; breathe deeply, clear your mind; and *relax.* If you spend ten minutes a day taking thirty- to sixty-second breaks between activities, you will feel less strained. I know you're busy, but you can afford to spend ten minutes a day de-stressing yourself. As a heart patient, you can't afford not to.
8. **Take charge of your worries.** Schedule some daily worry time—no more than fifteen to forty-five minutes—after which you promise to switch channels and direct your mental energies to another endeavor.

   Let's imagine you set aside half an hour in the morning to worry. Get paper and pen, sit down at a table, ask yourself these questions, and write down the answers:

   • What am I worried about?
   • How likely is this to happen?

- What's the worst that could happen?
- How will I cope in the immediate future if the worst does happen?
- What might be a long-term solution to this problem, or plan for dealing with it?
- What could I do *right now* that would help me worry a little less?

Listing your worries and analyzing your fantasy of the worst-case scenario will counteract the temptation to inflate worries into catastrophes, and doing something to quiet yourself will help you get through the day.

9. **Exercise.** Regular exercise helps you manage stress by:

- Lowering the level to which your stress can spike
- Enabling you to recover more quickly from a bout of stress
- Boosting your ability to activate the relaxation response
- Improving your self-confidence

10. **Avoid caffeine, nicotine, and too much simple sugar.** Coffee, tea, cigarettes, soft drinks, and candy all contain stimulants that fuel stress. Cut down on your consumption of these substances, and cut them out where you can.

11. **Straighten up your living and work spaces.** Mess brings stress; a tidy environment soothes.

12. **Become aware of noise pollution and silence it.** Turn off the television, radio, and stereo, doff your headphones, and discover why peace goes with quiet. What we hear affects muscle tension, blood pressure, and stress levels. Also, you cannot minimize aural stimuli easily the way you can visual stimuli; our sense of hearing is always on, even when we sleep. You must make a conscious choice to quiet your surroundings.

13. **Reach out to others.** Write a letter to a friend; better yet, pay him or her a visit. Being with people you enjoy is a potent way to lower stress and feel happier.

14. **Read for entertainment.** Make time to read books, journals, magazines, poetry, fiction, nonfiction—whatever entertains you that has nothing to do with your work or your worries. The point here is not just to read what you enjoy, but to read something that sweeps you away from the routines of your life.

15. **Associate with people who nurture you; avoid those who stir up hostile or competitive feelings.** Life is stressful enough. Don't make it worse by associating with people who make you angry or anxious. We all know people whose sense of humor thrives on put-downs or whose conversation dwells uncomfortably in the realm of the bleak and cynical. Spend as little time with these people as possible; they will sap your spirit and weaken your resolve to heal.

16. **Learn to laugh at yourself and admit your faults.** It will help you maintain proper perspective on your problems and keep you connected with others.

17. **Ask for and grant forgiveness.** There are no perfect people. We've all said and done things we regret. Don't live in guilty silence about these lapses; ask for forgiveness. You'll relieve your conscience as well as your stress level.

18. **Glance at yourself in a mirror from time to time** throughout the day to see if your face suggests that you are stressed, tired, angry, or worried. Then do something about what you see.

19. **Smile often.** Happiness is contagious. When you smile at others, they'll usually smile back, and it feels good.

20. **Don't argue when you know it would be pointless to do so.** Limit your battles to those you have a chance of winning. Conflict is stressful whether you win or lose, but losing is more stressful than winning.

21. **Resist the urge to lash out in anger.** When it comes to managing anger and conflict, it's better to speak up either before you reach the boiling point—when you're merely irritated but not yet infuriated—or, if you've already boiled over, to wait until you've cooled off a bit (see Chapter 8).

22. **Eat sensibly.** A heart-healthy diet also happens to be great for managing stress.

FINALLY, GET SOME SLEEP!

Sleep is a natural healer and restores your ability to cope. When you don't get adequate sleep, your worries seem worse than they really are (have you ever noticed that things always seem worse at night?). Sleep deprivation can interfere with concentration, mood, and body functions, and compromise your heart's ability to heal.

If your sleep patterns have changed, the stress or depression you're experiencing may be sleep-related. Talk with your doctor about your symptoms. In the meantime, here are a few tips to help you get a good night's sleep.

- Make your bedroom comfortable. Get a good mattress and make sure the temperature of the room is neither too warm nor too cool. If you and your partner disagree on the ideal bedroom temperature, compromise by using an extra blanket on one side of the bed or getting an electric blanket with two controls.

- If you have difficulty breathing when you lie down, try the following solutions:

- Elevate the head of the bed by placing its feet on wooden blocks between four and six inches tall.
- Lie atop a soft pillow that elevates your chest, shoulders, and head.
- Try using a vaporizer; warm, moist air makes breathing easier.
- Use any combination of the above.

- Avoid food, caffeine, alcohol, and smoking near bedtime.
- Don't nap in the afternoon or after dinner.
- Develop a nighttime routine:

  - Go to bed at the same time each night.
  - Awaken at the same time each morning.
  - Accustom yourself to doing the same things before bed each night.

- Exercise early in the day if possible; if not, leave at least four hours between your workout and bedtime.
- Use your bed and bedroom for sleeping (rather than watching television, catching up on work, and the like). If you don't fall asleep within thirty minutes, get out of bed, go to another room, and do something until you feel sleepy again.
- If you awaken earlier than usual, don't fret. Instead, relax yourself with pleasant thoughts, or the techniques you learned earlier, or both. If you don't fall back asleep, get out of bed and do something else until you feel sleepy again.
- Don't worry about not getting enough rest. Your body will let you fall asleep when you really need to.

If stress is the consequence of coping with change, managing stress is the act of summoning that which is unchanging within you. Managing stress is a personal, even intimate endeavor. It requires that you peel away your many layers until you see your true self, which glows in the core of your being. This true self thrives in the quiet knowledge of its essential nature, and you can know your nature only if you look inside without recoiling, discover what brings you peace, and gather it to you. Don't look to others for guidance here: what soothes your soul may rile someone else's, and what one person finds annoying may impart bliss to another. Neither should you attempt a temperamental makeover; if you're an intense, driven person, you probably won't mellow into a devil-may-care type no matter how many bubble baths you take. Try one way; if it doesn't work, try another. Pay attention to what makes you feel good, and do it more often. Trust yourself: you know what to do.

Chapter Seven

DEAL WITH DEPRESSION

(Most Heart Patients Get It; Why Should You Be Different?)

In his memoir *The Noonday Demon,* Andrew Solomon writes:

> To be creatures who love, we must be creatures who can despair at what we lose, and depression is the mechanism of that despair. When it comes, it degrades one's self and ultimately eclipses the capacity to give or receive affection. It is the aloneness within us made manifest, and it destroys not only connection to others but also the ability to be peacefully alone with oneself.[1]

The desolate landscape Solomon describes is familiar to anyone who has endured the anguish of depression. The numbing of feeling and sense of drifting beyond the reach of others can hobble even the hardiest spirit and erode the sturdiest sense of self. While depression summons many emotions—sadness, regret, and grief among them—the essence of depression is diminishment of feeling and weakening of will until all that remains is grim acceptance of an existence that only vaguely resembles a life.

Depression is an international epidemic. Between 10 and 14 million Americans and over 100 million people worldwide suffer from it. I mentioned earlier that as many as 75 percent of bypass patients wrestle with major depression after the procedure. About 30 percent of heart attack survivors struggle with major depression during long-term recovery, and between 40 and 65 percent experience at least sporadic depressed or anxious moods.[2]

If you wrestle with an occasional bout of the blues, you're not likely to suffer any long-term ill effects. Untreated depression is not only painful, however, it is hazardous to your heart. If you are living with depression and not getting help, you're not only increasing your odds of developing additional heart illness, you may also be complicating your recovery and hastening your death. Don't underestimate the gravity of this condition: a person who has had a heart attack, becomes depressed, and doesn't seek help is tripling—yes, *tripling*—the chance that he or she will die within six months.

DEPRESSION IS DANGEROUS

Most studies agree: *Depressed heart patients are more than twice as likely to require bypass surgery, suffer other heart-related complications, and have follow-up heart attacks than patients who are not depressed.* Here's what some of those studies found:

- Major depression can lead to early death for recovering heart attack patients.[3]

- For recent heart attack patients, depression is a more accurate predictor of future heart problems than severity of artery damage, high cholesterol levels, or cigarette smoking.[4]

- In a ten-year study of 230 first-time male and female heart attack patients younger than sixty-five, depression and lack of emotional support increased the risk of death from heart disease more powerfully than did marital stress, job stress, anxiety, or anger.[5]

- If you're over sixty, have high blood pressure (hypertension), are depressed, and aren't doing anything about it, you're more than doubling your risk of suffering a stroke or heart attack[6] or developing congestive heart failure.[7]

- Even if you don't have high blood pressure, depression increases your risk of dying from congestive heart failure (CHF).[8]

And you don't have to be paralyzed with sadness to be in danger: living with even mild depression increases your risk of death after a heart attack, according to a recent study at Johns Hopkins University. Researchers analyzed symptoms of depression in 285 heart attack survivors to measure the severity of their melancholy against their subsequent health problems. Here's what they found:

- Minimally depressed patients were *five times* as likely to die after their heart attacks as patients who were not depressed.

- Moderately depressed patients were *seven to eight times* as likely to die as those who were not depressed.

- Patients with high levels of depression were *eight to ten times* as likely to die as those who were not depressed.[9]

In other words, the more depressed you are, the higher your risk of dying after a heart attack, but living with even a low level of chronic depression significantly increases your risk of death if you've had a heart attack.

HOW DEPRESSION AFFECTS HEART HEALTH

Depression complicates your recovery in several ways. First, depressed people tend not to take very good care of themselves. When you're depressed, it's difficult to motivate yourself to exercise at all, let alone regularly, to eat well, or otherwise to take care of yourself. A haze of so-what thinking descends and clouds your view of the future; you think, *So what if I don't exercise? So what if I have a burger and fries? What's the big deal?*

Well, it *is* a big deal, and it *does* make a difference. The fact is, when you're depressed, you're more likely to choose unhealthy behaviors such as smoking, drinking, and gorging on foods that soothe you for the moment but hurt you in the long run.

Depressed heart patients also tend to abandon heart-healthy eating and exercise regimens and are less likely to participate in cardiac rehabilitation programs, take their medications as prescribed, and keep their doctors' appointments than nondepressed patients. And some scientists speculate that depressed patients recognize and respond to their symptoms more slowly than nondepressed patients, allowing the disease to progress further and reducing the impact of any medical care they may eventually receive.[10]

There also seems to be a connection between depressed mood and cardiac activity in ways that can complicate heart illness. For example:

- Depressed people—even if they don't have heart disease—have abnormal blood platelet activity and are more likely than those who are not depressed to develop clots in their arteries.[11]

- Depression prompts the brain to release stress hormones that can cause or complicate heart rhythm disturbances, or arrhythmias, of the sort that can lead to sudden cardiac death.[12]

- Depressed heart patients have more stress alarm responses (they activate their sympathetic nervous systems more frequently) but fewer calming responses (they activate their parasympathetic nervous systems less frequently) than nondepressed patients, increasing the likelihood that their stress will evolve into strain, and decreasing their chances of recovering fully from a heart attack.[13]

As if all this weren't enough, depression also has a corrosive effect on your attitude, weakening your resolve to change behaviors that could help you heal.

YOU DON'T HAVE TO BE DEPRESSED!

Now that I've told you the bad news, here's the great news: **Depression is curable.** That's right—it's curable. The new antidepressant medicines are safe for most heart patients and very effective at curing depression when you combine them with simple self-help techniques.

This is news because, for many years, doctors couldn't prescribe antidepressants for heart patients because the medications would worsen their heart conditions. The new antidepressants have changed all that. Physicians also have a better understanding of depression. After decades of viewing depression as a psychological condition, we have finally grasped that depression is a disease that manifests itself physically as well as psychologically. What we now know, and what *you* should know, is that:

- Depression is a medical condition.
- Depression is related to the brain through chemistry; to the mind through thought and behavior; and to the body through bodily changes.
- You can fight and triumph over depression by altering your brain chemistry (with medication), your depressive thought patterns (by learning new, more realistic ones), and your behaviors (by orchestrating your daily routines).
- Once your depression lifts, so do the health risks that descended with it.

It's a fact: in heart patients, depression correlates closely with physical functioning. A recent study followed a group of men and women out of the hospital after their heart attacks and into a cardiac rehab program and found that, regardless of age, changes in a patient's level of depression was one of the best indicators that his or her physical functioning would also change. The less depressed patients became, the higher they scored on physical exams.[14]

ARE YOU DEPRESSED?

This is not as simple a question as it sounds, as depression may be so much a part of your life that you don't even realize it's there. It's like an ancient gnarled oak that's always dominated your backyard: you can't even imagine the view without it, so you cease noticing it after a while; its existence seems inevitable. It's the same with depression; many people are convinced of the inevitability of their sadness. It's always been there; it feels like home.

That was the case with Jonas, a forty-nine-year-old social worker who had recently had quadruple bypass surgery after a heart attack two years earlier. In our first session, I learned that Jonas had been living in a committed partnership with Kurt, a fifty-one-year-old historian, for fourteen years, but that he had yet to come out to his family:

"This illness has been a bittersweet experience. The heart attack really got my attention—I mean, I was only forty-seven! It sounds like such a cliché, but it really woke me up to what's important—my life with Kurt, my family . . . and that's the bitter part. I've got two brothers and a sister whom I get along with, I guess, but I don't see them very often. I'm closest with my sister; she's been to visit Kurt and me, and she's fine with the fact that I'm gay. But my parents— my father was a minister, my mother worked part-time at the church. They're retired now, but if my father found out I was gay, it would kill him. He's eighty-five and he's got a heart condition, too, and I just cannot bring myself to tell him. I think my mother knows, but she's never said anything to me about it. And my brothers probably know, but they're kind of close with my dad, so I pretend to be the guy they think I am whenever I see them.

"That's the worst part—seeing my family. Even though Kurt and I have been together for fourteen years, my family still acts as if he's my roommate, so he never comes with me to family gatherings or celebrations. Christmas, Thanksgiving, Easter—we're always apart. Kurt's a good sport—he's had years of practice—but he's getting fed up with it.

"And I'm not feeling too good, either. I've been really down ever since the bypass. It's over two months now, but I can't shake it. I mean, I could die any time, and I'm still acting like a little boy, pretending to be someone I'm not.

"And now there's a crisis. My brother is getting married again, and I cannot bear the thought of going without Kurt. He's nursed me through a heart attack and bypass surgery; he's the closest person to me in this world. What should I do—stay away from my brother's wedding and offend my whole family? Leave Kurt home and make us both feel horrible? Or bring him and have my father drop dead of a heart attack when we walk in together?"

Jonas's depression was rooted in the conflict between his two selves: the one he showed his family, and his authentic self. Living an inauthentic life is a churning source of both stress and depression. It's like carrying out a self-imposed life sentence in a psychological witness protection program: you must live in eternal vigilance against anyone knowing the real you. In Jonas's case, this lack of authenticity had fostered a pervasive depression that limited his ability to see the options he had.

After several months of counseling, Jonas's depression became visible to him, as did the role that his double life was playing in it. I'd like to be able to tell you that he finally told his parents he was gay, fell into their arms, and received their unconditional acceptance, but that's not what happened. Jonas believed that the truth would devastate his father and ruin the end of his father's life, if not hasten it, so he chose not to confront him. But he did decide to take Kurt to the wedding, an action that bespoke a new commitment to living an authentic life. And that's the point: you can't deal with your depression if you don't know it's there. Once you know, you can do something.

SIGNS OF DEPRESSION

It's likely you're depressed if you notice changes in your mood, manner of thinking, behavior patterns, and bodily functions that last more than three or four weeks.[15]

The **moods** associated with depression transcend sadness. In fact, some people suffer from depression and aren't aware of it because they associate depression with feelings of despondency, and they just don't feel that way. Psychiatrist Peter V. Rabins says that at least a third of his clinically depressed patients claim they don't feel sad or blue. He also says that men are especially likely to deny being depressed because they are embarrassed by their symptoms.[16] So be aware that sadness is only one feeling that's associated with depression; you may also feel anxious, angry, melancholy, irritable, or a general malaise, as if everything is wrong, nothing is right, and you cannot find a place for yourself in the world. When you're depressed, you may feel as if you're in a permanent bad mood and lose interest in things that usually bring you pleasure. Many depressed people feel that something terrible is about to happen and are perpetually anxious. You may feel so hopeless and helpless that thoughts of suicide creep into your consciousness.

Depressed thinking manifests itself as a predominantly pessimistic point of view, especially about yourself and your situation. Depressed people have difficulty seeing any good in themselves, their past, or their future.

When you're depressed, your thoughts brim with images and self-talk that persuade you that, before the illness, your life was wonderful and now that you're sick, it will never be the same. You may have trouble concentrating and remembering things because you're preoccupied with thinking about the bleakness of your situation. You may also find yourself procrastinating more than usual because your pessimism has eroded your confidence in your ability to make good decisions.

When you're depressed, you may notice a change in your **behavior patterns,** even something as simple as your ability to carry out everyday activities. The thought of going to the market may be so daunting that you end up eating mayonnaise sandwiches for four days. Or you may sit in your living room watching the front yard go to seed because you cannot will yourself to drag the lawn mower out of the garage. Depression can pin you to the sofa, writhing in guilt and anxiety about all you should be doing while feeling utterly incapable of doing anything.

Depression also affects **bodily functions.** Some people lose interest in food when they're depressed and grow thin; others obsess about food and put on weight. Depression can also interfere with sleep patterns; as with eating, the changes can go either way. Many depressed people have trouble falling asleep or staying asleep, or awaken several hours earlier than they normally do, cannot go back to sleep, and begin their days at four A.M. Others have the opposite reaction, feel constantly fatigued, and sleep as many as twelve or more hours a day. In either case, depression usually makes you feel depleted and lethargic, regardless of how much you sleep. Other bodily changes associated with depression include loss of interest in sex, dry mouth, constipation, and vague, unexplained pains in different parts of the body.

To help you figure out whether you are depressed, I have reprinted below a list of symptoms adapted from the *Diagnostic and Statistical Manual of Mental Disorders IV* (or *DSM–IV* for short), the standard by which medical professionals interpret and define psychological conditions.[17] Read through the following statements and check any that apply to you:

____ I feel hopeless all the time, as if there's no way to solve my problems.

____ I used to enjoy doing many things, but they don't interest me any more.

____ I can't seem to feel pleasure. My sex drive is down, and I generally have a passive, so-what attitude about my life, as if nothing matters anymore.

____ My appetite is going wild—I can't stop eating, and I've put on a lot of weight.

___ My appetite has disappeared; food doesn't interest me any more. I've lost weight, which I guess is good, but people tell me I'm starting to look too skinny.

___ I can't sleep normally anymore. (Check this one if you have insomnia [inability to fall asleep], or disrupted sleep [difficulty staying asleep], or are sleeping more than usual.)

___ I feel nervous and jumpy all the time.

___ I feel tired all the time, even when I've had a good night's sleep. I just don't have any energy; it's as if my muscles weigh hundreds of pounds.

___ I feel guilty and inadequate, as if nothing I do will ever measure up.

___ I'm having trouble thinking clearly and concentrating; I forget lots of things, and it's hard for me to make decisions.

___ I keep thinking about death, about what a relief it would be to be done with everything. I sometimes think I might want to end my life.

If you checked five or more of these symptoms and have been experiencing the symptoms more often than not for the past several weeks, you may be suffering from clinical depression. This kind of depression is dangerous to your heart and requires medical attention.

CONQUERING DEPRESSION

You *can* beat depression! Here are five steps to help you do it:

1. Seek medical help.
2. Manage depressive thinking.
3. Change depressive behaviors.
4. Attend to your relationships.
5. Consider counseling.

Let's go over them one by one.

1. SEEK MEDICAL HELP.

I place this one first because you must accept that clinical depression—the kind that afflicts you with the symptoms just discussed—is a *medical* condition, not a state of mind. No amount of self-talk, exercise, or friendly encouragement will cure major depression because neither personality flaws, laziness, nor lack of willpower causes it.

Clinical depression results when the brain's chemicals are out of balance,

---

IT *COULD* BE SOMETHING ELSE

It is possible to experience classic symptoms of depression and be suffering from something else. Alcohol abuse, personality disorders, sleep apnea (a serious disorder in which a person repeatedly stops breathing while sleeping), and thyroid problems can all cause symptoms that resemble those of depression. Also, heart patients sometimes suffer brain-related blood vessel damage that may cause depression (see Chapter 2). Finally, some medications prescribed for heart ailments may have depressive side effects (see the Appendix). If you are experiencing symptoms you suspect may be masquerading as depression, consult your physician.

---

which is why taking an antidepressant medication is the most effective way to fight it. If you don't like the idea of taking medication, you're not alone: I've had many patients cringe when they hear me talk about it. They tell me they don't want to take anything, they don't even like swallowing an aspirin, they've always been strong-minded and determined, they want to solve their own problems. I listen, I tell them I understand their concerns, and then I tell them what I'll tell you now: if you want to solve your own problems, you'll have a much better chance of doing it if you take an antidepressant. And you're more likely to make the most of the medication's benefits if you and your loved ones understand why you need it, how it works, and that it is safe.

Why Use Medications?

Antidepressants are not addictive. They work gradually and gently and do not cause a high or buzz of any sort. What they do is rectify the ebb and flow of chemicals in the brain.

A good way to understand clinical depression is to think of it as a temporary botching of the brain's chemical and electrical activity. Picture your brain as an electrical command center housing billions of nerve cells, or neurons, whose endings are separated by minuscule gaps called synapses. The brain controls your thinking and emotions through the lightning-fast leaping of impulses from one neuron to the next. These impulses are the brain's messages to your body, and travel down a neuron's shaft, leap over the synapse to the next neuron, then speed to parts of the brain that enable you to think, make decisions, recall memories, control your moods, and so on.

To help a message sprint from one neuron to the next, the sending neuron ending secretes a chemical called a neurotransmitter into the synapse. This tiny pool of fluid temporarily connects the endings, hastening the impulse's journey across the synapse and onward to another part of the brain. Once the impulse clears the synapse, the receiving neuron ending absorbs the chemical, clearing the synapse and readying it for the next impulse.

When secretion and absorption of the neurotransmitter don't work properly, the brain sometimes fires an impulse over and over again. This makes it hard for a person to move past bothersome thoughts, think clearly, and control emotions. The result is clinical depression.

Clearing the Synapses

The body has ways of correcting its chemistry. For example, when you exercise, enjoy a good laugh, or delight in physical affection, whether it's sexual relations or a good long hug, your brain releases chemicals that soothe and relax you, at least for a while. When you're not depressed, this soothing effect can linger for hours. But clinical depression short-circuits the lingering effect: as you leave the gym or disengage from the hug, the depression crashes back down around your ears. This is where an antidepressant makes such a big difference: by adjusting the brain's ability to control the secretion and flow of its chemicals.

If you're a depressed heart patient, there has never been a greater abundance of medications to help you than there is today. More prescriptions are written for antidepressants than for any other class of drugs except heart medications. And more and more people are taking them: in 2001, 7.1 million Americans took some form of antidepressant, 700,000 more than the year before.[18] In fact, some of the newer ones, known as selective serotonin reuptake inhibitors, or SSRIs, have proven not only to treat depression safely but also to reduce the clustering of blood platelets in arteries, hindering the formation of blockages and improving cardiac functioning after a heart attack.[19]

Another, even newer variety, known as selective serotonin *and norepinephrine* reuptake inhibitors, or SSNRIs, acts upon both serotonin and norepinephrine simultaneously. Scientists are experimenting with SSNRIs in the belief that zapping two neurotransmitters at once may provide patients with more effective relief than targeting only one.

For the most part, the newer antidepressants are safe for heart patients but

> **If you are taking an antiarrhythmic or beta-blocker medication, be sure to alert all your doctors before starting an antidepressant. Antidepressants can interact with cardiac drugs in ways that complicate their effects.**

do have some cardiovascular side effects: they may affect heart rhythms (causing the heart to beat faster or slower); cause vasoconstriction (whereby blood vessels contract, limiting their ability to deliver blood to various body parts), or they may interact with other medications. For example, at higher dosages, venlafaxine (Effexor) increases both blood pressure and heart rate by up to four beats per minute.[20] This doesn't mean you shouldn't take an antidepressant; but it does mean you should never take a medication—even one prescribed by your physician—without discussing with him or her its possible cardiac side effects. Also, when consulting physicians other than your cardiologist, remember to remind them that you are a heart patient.

Don't Take the Quick-and-Easy Way Out—It Isn't

Depression is painful, and it's tempting to use alcohol, caffeine, or nicotine for a rapid dose of relief. Although they may supply some nearly instant gratification, the buzz will wear off and your depression will return, often with complications, since they are addictive. Alcohol, after all, is a depressant, so it cannot elevate your mood.

Depressed cardiac patients must be especially wary of overusing alcohol because of its corrosive effect on heart tissue. Research suggests that one out of four hospital patients and one out of five people who visit outpatient facilities are alcohol-dependent,[21] with many of them not even realizing it. They know they like to have a few drinks, but they don't know that they have grown dependent on those drinks to feel comfortable in their own skins. Nor do they know that alcohol is contributing to their depression.

Be honest with yourself: is there a chance you might be overusing alcohol and relying on it to get you through? Even if you think not, take thirty seconds to answer these four questions:[22]

___ Yes ___ No Have you ever felt you should cut down on your drinking?

___ Yes ___ No Have people ever annoyed you by criticizing your
drinking?

___ Yes ___ No Have you ever felt bad or guilty about your drinking?

___ Yes ___ No Have you ever had a drink first thing in the morning—
an "eye-opener"—to steady your nerves or get rid of a
hangover?

According to J. A. Ewing, M.D., an addictions expert at the University of
North Carolina, if you answered yes to two or more of the questions, there's
an 85 to 95 percent chance that you are either overusing alcohol or dependent on it.[23] If you think you might be overusing alcohol or nonprescrip-
tion drugs, talk to your doctor or another health care professional. If you're
considering using an antidepressant, it's especially important to be honest
with your doctor about how much alcohol you use. Why? Again—because
alcohol is a depressant and can interfere with the positive effects of antidepressant medication.

Get the Right Medication and Stay on It

Antidepressants help relieve depression between 60 and 70 percent of the
time, especially when the person taking them also goes for counseling and
uses self-help antidepression techniques. But many patients sabotage their
opportunity to conquer depression by:

- Taking the wrong medication
- Taking the wrong dosage of the medication
- Stopping the medication too soon

TAKING THE WRONG MEDICATION

Not all antidepressants are the same, and they affect different people in different ways, both in terms of how they operate on the condition and the
side effects they may cause. For example, there may be two antidepressants
that are right for you, but one may make you feel sedated while the other
may energize you. If your doctor prescribes an antidepressant, find out
everything you can about it: its generic and brand names, its manufacturer,
how much your dosage will be, how you may expect to feel when you're taking it, how long it is likely to be before you feel better, and possible side effects, both common and uncommon. You are more likely to stick with and
benefit from a medication if you know what to expect when you're taking it.
(See the Appendix for a list of commonly prescribed antidepressants.)

If you are already taking an antidepressant, pay attention to changes in both your mood and bodily functions. If, for example, you started having stomach discomfort at about the same time you started taking an antidepressant, it is likely the medication is causing the problem. Call your physician, describe your symptoms, and ask him or her if a different drug might be better for you.

Taking the Wrong Dosage of the Medication

While physicians do their best to prescribe appropriate dosages, they don't always get it right the first time. Also, when prescribing a medication that's new to a patient, doctors will sometimes start with a low dosage so they can monitor the patient's reaction to the drug while its effects are still relatively mild.

How can you tell if you're taking the correct dosage of a medication? Once again, you must pay attention to how you're feeling. If you have been taking an antidepressant for several months and aren't feeling better, speak to your doctor; you might need a higher dosage. It also works the other way: if you are experiencing unusual bodily or psychological changes, they could be the result of taking too high a dosage. For example, if you start feeling excessively fatigued or are unable to concentrate and think clearly, you may need a lower dosage of your antidepressant.

Stopping the Medication Too Soon

I cannot count the patients I've counseled who have started an antidepressant, begun feeling better, stopped taking the medication, and then come to see me because they're feeling blue and don't know why. The reason is, of course, that they stopped taking the medication as soon as they started feeling better, which is almost always too soon.

Most patients feel their depression begin to lift two to four weeks after starting an antidepressant. As their mood improves, many continue taking the medication for another month or so, and then stop, believing they're cured.

This is a mistake. For an antidepressant to have a lasting effect, you must continue to take it well after you have started to feel better, perhaps even indefinitely. In 2003, the British journal *The Lancet* published research by scientists at Oxford University who analyzed thirty years of studies and found that patients who stopped taking their antidepressants were twice as likely to become depressed again as those who stayed on them.[24]

Taking an antidepressant is like taking an antibiotic: you must take a full course of treatment in order for it to work. When you have a sinus infection, your doctor prescribes a ten-day course of an antibiotic (some of the newer ones require a three- to five-day course). Even though your headache might abate and your nose stop running after the first few doses, it's important to finish the prescription or the infection will probably return. That's because the antibiotic must build to a high enough level in the body to kill the infection and not just relieve the symptoms.

It's the same with an antidepressant. Just because your depressive symptoms have abated doesn't mean the medication has adequately adjusted your brain chemistry. You must continue taking the medication well beyond the time that you begin to feel better until you *become* better.

2. MANAGE DEPRESSIVE THINKING.

The second step in conquering depression is to manage depressive thinking. When you are depressed, your mind scans for thoughts that bother you, seizes upon them, and presses them into your consciousness like cloves in a holiday ham. Thoughts of failure, loss, and even suicide can fix in your mind and resist even the most spirited attempts to dislodge them.

You already know how dangerous it is for heart patients to indulge in pessimistic thinking, so I won't go into it again here. But I will tell you that managing your thinking—deliberately forging positive, hopeful thoughts from negative, cynical ones—is a potent weapon against the paralysis of depression.

Whenever I tell patients about the importance of managing their thinking, I think about Nora. Nora first came to see me on an October day as gray as her spirits. A dignified African American, she looked older than her seventy years and wrung her hands throughout our session.

Nora's life had been in turmoil for over a year, since that December when, as she said, the bomb dropped on her happy little life. As usual, she and her husband, Louis, had served Christmas dinner to their three daughters, two sons-in-law, and four grandchildren. Not as usual, Louis had surprised Nora by reserving a suite with a view at a high-priced mountain resort and taking her away for a romantic New Year's weekend. As Nora described it, they had just returned home and she was unpacking the party favors from her suitcase when Louis came into the room wearing a shirt she didn't recognize and a solemn expression:

"We had just gotten back and Louis looks at me, all sad and sincere, and says he's in love with another woman and he's leaving. I just stood there, stunned, with those damned noisemakers in my hand. He'd planned the whole thing— the fancy weekend, telling me how much I meant to him . . . I swear, I must

have stood there for an hour. I never did empty his suitcase; I think he just closed it again and took it with him when he left the next day.

"My life became a nightmare, only I couldn't wake up. If it weren't for my girls and their families, I would not have made it. I know that for a fact because I was thinking about doing away with myself and they're the ones who convinced me I had something to live for. Then, six months later, another bomb exploded, this time in my chest. I was in the hospital for two weeks. The day I came home, I sank into a real depression. I kept hearing my own voice in my head, scolding me for being so stupid.

"Then a miracle happened: Louis came back. His fifty-year-old girlfriend decided she wasn't ready to marry a senior citizen, so there he was, back in my arms. He couldn't have been more patient and loving. He nursed me through the next six months; he never left my side. I remember thanking God one night for blessing me with heart disease because it brought my husband back. That's how distorted my thinking was.

"It was about eight months after the heart attack and I was getting much stronger when—big surprise!—Louis left again, this time for good.

"Life goes on. The kids help a lot. And the rehab program—it's helping me deal with my fear of this illness. You know, I used to walk around all the time picturing my heart about to explode. But in rehab I learned how to shift the image when it comes into my head; now I picture my heart beating strong and steady.

"Sometimes I get blue, wishing Louis were with me. But then I think, at least I'm here, holding the grandchildren and watching them grow. And I made myself a promise: No more rushing. I spent most of my life in a hurry, putting everyone else first. Now I think about myself more. I take life slower so I can savor it more. And it was the heart attack, not the divorce, that made me change."

Nora's challenge—to divert her thoughts from negative pathways and reroute them toward hopeful ones—is one that every heart patient faces. Hopeless, negative thoughts are the stuff of which depression is made. These thoughts do not represent the truth about you, your life, or the people around you. They are thoughts born of distortion and despair, and they no more represent reality than a fish-eye camera lens does.

Is It Depression or Grief?

Every heart patient endures losses. Heart illness shatters a person's illusions of immortality and perfect health, along with the ability to enjoy unrestricted activity and the fantasy of living without fear. Grief is a natural response to such losses and can darken a heart patient's life in ways that mimic depression, sometimes making it difficult to tell the two apart.

Grief and depression overlap in many ways: both can sadden you, sap your energy, and cause you to obsess about your emotional distress. But they are different: grief passes more quickly than depression and tends to lift, however temporarily, when other people offer comfort. Depression, on the other hand, seldom lifts through the ministrations of others. Also, while grief and depression can both cause obsessive thoughts, a grieving person tends to think about the loss while a depressed person focuses inward, on feelings of worthlessness.

Grief passes with time; depression usually doesn't. If your anguish becomes severe and you begin to think about harming yourself, **seek professional help immediately.** You cannot trust yourself to think clearly when you're feeling this low, and you must promise yourself, right now, that you will get a physician or therapist to help you through.

3. Change Depressive Behaviors.

The third step in conquering depression involves managing your behaviors. Remember the "imagine it, act it, become it" technique from Chapter 5? This technique operates on the principle that if you can imagine an attitude you can act as if you feel that way, and if you act that way long enough, you will become that way. When you're immobilized with despair, you can use this technique to remind yourself of how you behave when you feel better.

The technique works because it asks you to change your behavior rather than your thinking, which is easier to do, especially when you're depressed. "Don't worry, be happy" won't be high on your hit parade when you can't find the strength to look at a newspaper. But you *can* force yourself to get dressed, comb your hair, go out and buy a newspaper, and make the effort to read it. You don't have to *feel* like doing something to do it; you just have to *will* yourself to do it.

You'll recall that the trick is to stick with the new behavior, especially in the early stage when it feels out of joint with your thinking. If you wait until you feel better before resuming your life, you are likely to grow even more deeply depressed. Many of my patients have used this technique and you can, too.

Here's how to start. Each day, whether you feel like it or not, do at least one thing from each of the following categories:

EXERCISE HELPS!

Regular exercise is a **must** for any depressed heart patient. When you work out, you counteract the physical and psychological causes of depression and improve your heart health as well. If you participate in a structured, exercise-based cardiac rehabilitation program, your depression **will** absolutely, positively diminish.[25]

- **Follow through with some of your duties and obligations.** These might include caring for your children or grandchildren, showing up at your job (on time and able to work), attending a rehab session, or performing everyday tasks such as bathing, dressing, going for a haircut, or buying groceries.
- **Do some things that will give you a sense of achievement.** These are chores and activities whose completion would normally give you a feeling of satisfaction or pride. You might tidy a messy closet, fix a leaky faucet, learn how to program the DVD player, clean out the garage, walk fifteen minutes longer than you planned to, or take your shoe boxes of snapshots and arrange them in albums.
- **Do at least one thing that would normally bring you pleasure, even if you don't feel like it.** This is a necessity, not a luxury, and can be anything you used to enjoy when you were feeling better but can't seem to enjoy now. What you choose depends on who you are: do a crossword puzzle, go out to a movie, sit down at the piano or pick up the guitar, play a game with the kids, go to lunch with a friend, or spend an hour watching your favorite talk show. It doesn't matter what you do as long as you do something that reminds you of what used to make you feel good.

Plan Your Day—Don't Wing It

When I counsel depressed patients, I tell them not to leave their schedules to chance. It's better to put pen to paper (or stylus to screen) and plan what you are going to do than to let it take care of itself (it rarely does). Get a pocket-size date book with enough space to jot down a full day's activities. Be specific; it's not enough to note that you'll be out all morning. Instead, note that from ten until eleven you'll be dropping off dry cleaning and picking up groceries; from eleven to twelve you'll be at the post office (leave extra time—there's always a line); and from twelve to one-thirty you'll be at Seven Brothers Pizzeria having lunch with Stan. Dividing your day into segments, each with a goal, prevents the hours ahead from looming as a vacant, lonely eternity. Remember: when you're depressed, you fill your time—and your mind—with depressive thoughts and images. Giving yourself small assignments structures your thinking as well as your time.

When you're feeling low, try to avoid:

- Being alone for long periods of time
- Listening to sad music, reading sad stories, and watching sad movies or television programs
- Weeping excessively without distracting yourself or involving yourself in an activity
- Getting angry, especially at family members who are trying to help you
- Blaming yourself or others for your moodiness
- Giving in to bad moods by indulging in self-pity
- Medicating yourself with alcohol, cigarettes, food, or drugs

4. ATTEND TO YOUR RELATIONSHIPS.

The fourth step in conquering depression is attending to your relationships. When you're depressed, it's natural to turn inward and become so involved in yourself that you disconnect from the people around you. It's particularly easy to do this when the people around you are the people who love you most, and are trying to hide their feelings in deference to yours.

It's crucial to remember that members of your family and recovery team worry about you when you're depressed, even if they don't show it. Some may try to cheer you up with small talk or offer advice, only to grow frustrated at their powerlessness to banish your blues. You may grow irritated with their efforts, snap at them, and then feel guilty about your outburst. Or you may withdraw further into your shell, rebuking even the gentlest attempts to coax you out.

In short, it is important that you show the people you love that you're aware your depression is affecting them. You don't have to feel guilty; depression is a medical condition, after all. It makes no more sense to feel guilty about being depressed than it does to castigate your character for having the flu. But you should take the initiative to tell your loved ones that you know you're not yourself these days, and you're grateful to them for standing by you. Here are some suggestions:

- "I'm sorry I've been so depressed lately. I know I'm not acting like myself."
- "I know I haven't been interested in sex for a while and that you're upset about it. I miss you, too. But I feel dead inside. I know that this will pass. I do love you, and I hope you can understand."
- "I know I'm not much fun to be around lately, and I'm sorry. Please forgive me if I've been unkind; I didn't mean to hurt your feelings."

You also need to let your family and friends know that you need their support. It helps if you can explain what is happening to you. You might try saying something like this:

- "I appreciate your taking the time to listen to me. I want you to know that I'm fighting depression. I'm getting help, and I believe I'll be better soon. But I'm feeling pretty low right now, and I'm grateful for your patience and support."

When They Disapprove of Your Course of Treatment

Some friends and family members might express concern about your taking antidepressant medication and caution you about possible health threats and side effects. Others might press you to transcend your depression with willpower and positive thinking alone. Still others may disapprove of counseling, citing therapy as a crutch for the weak of will and exhorting you to be strong enough to find your own answers.

These folks may mean well, but they're ill informed. It might be helpful to have them read this chapter so they can better understand what you're dealing with and what your treatment plan involves.

5. CONSIDER COUNSELING.

The fifth step in conquering depression—one that enhances the potency of the other four—is going for counseling. A skilled therapist can help you and your family both as individuals and as a unit. A psychiatrist, psychologist, social worker, or psychiatric nurse would be a good person to consider as a counselor. Ask your physician to recommend someone whom he or she knows to be experienced at counseling cardiac patients and their families. Your health insurance carrier should also be able to recommend a roster of mental health professionals whose services are covered under your plan.

IN CONCLUSION

If you have heart disease, chances are good that at some point you have felt melancholy or depressed (or you will in the future). But you don't have to live that way. With medication, counseling, and the will to fight back, **you can and will conquer depression. Coping with this condition may be the most important step you take in your journey toward recovery.**

Remember—if you become depressed:

- See a physician and get medical help.
- Don't let it flatten you; *fight back*.
- Structure your time; create a daily schedule and stick to it.
- Exercise regularly.
- If you feel stuck, vary your routine.
- Enjoy simple, healthy pleasures.
- Start small.
- Distract yourself from depressive feelings by avoiding depressive behaviors. Don't wallow in self-pity.
- Dissipate pessimistic thoughts by channeling your mind toward optimistic ones.
- Think about all the things you're thankful for, write them down, and post the list in open view.
- Ask family members and friends for comfort and support, and offer some in return.
- If your pain becomes severe and you begin to have thoughts of harming yourself, call someone, tell him or her how you're feeling, and ask for help.
- Go for counseling.
- Have courage; press on. You *will* feel better.

Chapter Eight

DEFUSE YOUR ANGER
BEFORE IT KILLS YOU

*Speak when you are angry and you will make
the best speech you will ever regret.*

—AMBROSE BIERCE [1]

Anger isn't healthy for anyone, but for a recovering heart patient, getting good and angry is like playing Russian roulette: maybe nothing will happen but, if it does, it could be explosive. If you have heart illness, a bout of anger more than doubles the chances that you'll suffer a heart attack within two hours of the episode.[2] And, unlike depression, which some patients say they cannot relate to, everyone knows what it's like to be angry.

Everyone has a memory, vivid and tinged with red, of when he or she lost control and got really angry. (Some of us have even more than one.) It may have happened at work, or at home, or standing in line at the bank. Perhaps you directed your rage at your kids, or the person with whom you share your life, or the hapless retail clerk who informed you that your order actually hadn't come in after you fought rush-hour traffic to get to the store after work. No doubt you had a right to be angry; you did the right thing, and you expect others to do the right thing, too. Only they seldom do, and you're left to deal with their incompetence, insensitivity, and stupidity.

Behavioral psychologists, who spend their lives studying this kind of thing, say that anger is the emotion hardest to control.[3] And it's no wonder; there isn't much incentive lately to keep your temper when so many of us are losing it for a living: alleged adults pummel one another on talk shows, rap musicians growl venomous lyrics at angry young fans, and political commentators lob verbal grenades at one another and call it news analysis. Popular culture (not to mention TV ratings) thrives on public displays of bad manners, ill-temper, and rage, so why should any of us even examine our cynicism and anger, let alone try to control them?

Because they're hurtful at best and fatal at worst. A landmark cardiology study determined that if *any* of the following descriptions apply to you, you may be suffering from a life-threatening condition: [4]

- Do relatively minor mistakes by others irritate or anger you, and do you find such mistakes hard to overlook?
- Do you frequently look for flaws in people and situations and fixate on what might go wrong?
- Are you often unable or unwilling to laugh at things that other people find humorous?
- Are you overly proud of your ideals and standards, and do you revel in telling others about them whether or not they ask?
- Do you tend to believe that most people cannot be trusted and that they are generally motivated by self-interest?
- Do you feel contemptuous of others?
- Do you regularly steer the conversation toward what is wrong with the world, the current administration, the older and younger generations, the poor, the rich, immigrants, corporate America, and anyone who isn't you?
- Do you pepper your speech with obscenities?
- Is it hard for you to compliment or congratulate others with sincere good will?

If these characteristics sound all too familiar, the life-threatening condition you may have is Type A behavior pattern. According to cardiologist Meyer Friedman and his colleagues at the Recurrent Coronary Prevention Project in San Francisco, failure to control any of these tendencies can fuel free-floating hostility, the most toxic component of the Type A syndrome, which every heart patient should be wary of. [5]

THE HEART OF THE MATTER

In the early 1980s, Friedman and his team coined a new term—"Type A behavior pattern"—to describe a complex of traits that, when they coalesce in an individual, form a coping style that may be hazardous to his or her health. The research began earlier, long before mind-body medicine was a household term—in 1957, to be precise—when Friedman's team conducted a study of forty accountants and discovered, to their surprise, that the accountants' blood cholesterol and clotting activity rose dangerously during tax time. Friedman and colleagues realized they were onto something—that a psychological factor such as stress could affect the chemistry and activity of the cardiovascular system. They pressed on with the research and, over the years, determined that Type A behavior pattern, or TABP, was as significant a risk factor for developing heart illness (or complicating it further) as hypertension, elevated cholesterol, and smoking.[6]

Type A behavior pattern is that hard-driving style of living that involves a combination of the following behaviors:

- Relentless attempts to accomplish more and more in less and less time (taking on more work responsibilities or social obligations than you can realistically meet)
- Constant rushing (speaking, driving, and moving more quickly than others, also known as hurry sickness)
- Competitiveness (measuring your worth by comparing yourself to others and attempting to outdo them)
- Focusing excessively on work and "success" (placing undue weight on your accomplishments in the workplace and the imagined admiration of others)
- Multitasking, which manifests itself as a tendency to do and think about more than one thing at a time (talking to a client on the phone while you mouth instructions to your assistant and scan stock prices on your computer)
- Perfectionism (striving for perfection, which you can never achieve, rather than excellence, which you can)
- Hypervigilance (keeping your eyes and ears piqued for any suggestion of a problem)
- Relating to others in a controlling way (acting in ways calculated to manipulate others' behavior)
- Hostility (an ongoing attitude that cultivates opportunities to feel and express dissatisfaction and anger)

No one (not even you) exhibits all these characteristics all the time. While you may recognize some of these behaviors as your own, it's likely that only certain situations or people inspire you to respond this way. That said, however, even a few of these behaviors can interact to increase your risk of suffering a cardiac event.[7] For example, people who are chronically rushing may overreact to situations that force them to slow down, such as having to wait in a long line or for a slow-moving mate when they want to leave the house.

Anger also impairs a person's ability to think clearly by diminishing cognitive processes such as memory, creativity, and concentration. When we get angry, our thinking shifts into a mode that heightens our perceptions of bad things, mutes the good ones, and impels us to treat assumptions—usually negative ones—as if they were facts. In these circumstances, frustrations quickly brew into hostility and hostility can escalate into calamity. That's what happened to Nelson.

Nelson was fifty-six years old, with a shock of brown hair that always looked a little disheveled and in need of a trim, wire-rimmed glasses, and a permanent smirk that often had me wondering if he were about to tell me a joke or tell me off. A technical writer, Nelson had relocated to North Carolina from Pittsburgh when his employer, an electronics firm, moved its corporate headquarters. He hated the move and spoke incessantly of how it had ruined his life. Interestingly, he never mentioned how his wife and three children—aged seventeen, fifteen, and thirteen—felt about it.

"I know how I like things, and I do what I can to make them that way," he said at our first session. "It took me most of the eighteen years I lived in Pittsburgh to find people who did things right. I had a decent health club, a fairly honest mechanic, a good dry cleaner, I found a guy who gave a terrific haircut at a fair price—the whole deal. I'm not saying these folks were perfect, but they were the best in town." (According to Yvonne, Nelson's wife, he used to complain bitterly about the incompetents in Pittsburgh, too.)

"And then I'm forced to move to this cow town. I tell you, the longer I live here, the more I'm convinced that the heart attack actually killed me and I've been sent to hell."

One day at work, Nelson was struck with what he figured was intense indigestion. He felt sick enough to visit the nurse, who took one look at him and called the paramedics. Nelson became furious, bombarding her with language I cannot repeat here. At the hospital, Nelson was diagnosed with acute myocardial infarction and three of his arteries were found to be partially blocked with atherosclerosis. His cardiologist ordered more tests before scheduling bypass surgery and in the meantime sent Nelson to rehab.

If you think Nelson sent flowers to the nurse, you're wrong. Instead, he arrived at rehab royally ticked off: "I knew that moving here would kill me! Now I'm stuck here, surrounded by doctors and nurses young enough to be my kids, saying, 'How're y'all feelin' today, hon?'"

I remember Nelson for many reasons, all of them sad. After he'd been in rehab for a couple of months, I witnessed a scene that haunts me years later. Mary and I were waiting in line to buy popcorn at the movies one evening when a ruckus broke out toward the front of the line. A middle-aged man was in the throes of a temper tantrum, head thrust forward, veins pulsing in his neck, cursing a college kid who had bumped into him and spilled his popcorn. The kid kept trying to apologize but the man would have no part of it. The scene ended abruptly when the man, face aflame, stalked off, cursing the stupid kid and the stupid theater. A moment later, a woman and three teenagers left the line and, with downcast eyes, followed him out. Only then did I realize the man was Nelson. His face and demeanor were so distorted and grotesque that I had not recognized him.

But that's not the worst of it. Nine weeks later, Nelson collapsed at work with a second massive heart attack. This time he didn't make it.

Of all the Type A factors, unchecked hostility has proven the most deadly, causing healthy people to develop heart illness and leading heart patients toward early death: [8]

- A study of ischemia—a condition resulting when the heart needs more oxygenated blood than its clogged arteries can deliver—determined that anger triggered more episodes than any other physical or mental activity, including smoking. [9]

- In a remarkable experiment, heart patients were asked to engage in a role-playing exercise and defend themselves against shoplifting charges, ride an exercise bicycle, do an arithmetic problem in their heads, and, finally, recall an event from the previous six months that still angered or frustrated them when they thought about it. Researchers monitored the patients' hearts throughout each task.

  The results? For 40 percent of the patients, simply recalling the upsetting event affected their hearts most radically, temporarily inhibiting the amount of blood they could pump—more than riding an exercise bike!—even though the patients said the anger and frustration they experienced in recalling the event *were less than half as intense as the original feelings.* [10]

- A hostile or angry reaction increases stress hormones such as norepinephrine, elevates fat levels in the blood, and heightens your physical reactions across the board. Let's say you're stuck in a traffic jam on the way to the airport and you arrive breathlessly at the check-in desk only to learn that the flight is overbooked, they've given away your seat, and the next flight they can put you on doesn't leave for three hours. Now you'll miss your connection, along with an important dinner meeting. Your breath comes faster, your heart starts to pound, and you want to throttle the attendant who you assume gave your seat to some jerk flying standby who couldn't care less which flight he got on. While your main sensations are of mounting rage and moisture in your armpits, other things are happening that you can't feel: norepinephrine is flowing into your system, slowing the removal of fat from the blood and crowding it with a surplus of red cells, a process called "sludging." This can choke off hundreds of tiny blood vessels for as long as twelve hours. (Incidentally, this is why some researchers warn that eating high-fat meals when you're angry can trigger a heart attack or even sudden death.) [11]

- Anger experts Redford and Virginia Williams warn that for the chronically hostile person, "getting angry is like taking a small dose of some slow-acting poison—arsenic, for example—every day of your life." [12] Compared to anger, arsenic sounds downright tame: *an outburst of anger doubles your risk of having a heart attack for two hours after the episode.* [13]

- Chronically hostile people, similarly to those who are chronically depressed, usually don't take good care of themselves. They tend to consume more caffeine, nicotine, alcohol, and calories and exercise less, sleep less, and even floss their teeth less frequently than more agreeable folks. [14] They also seem to have a self-destructive streak, as they are more likely than less hostile people to drive recklessly or while under the influence of alcohol or drugs.

CHANGE YOUR BEHAVIOR, SAVE YOUR LIFE

As always, I have very good news:

1. It *is* possible for even the oldest dog to learn to change its ways.
2. Doing so can save your life.

The most impressive proof comes from the tireless Dr. Friedman and his team, which, after identifying Type A behavior pattern (TABP), set out to compare the effectiveness of two different treatments for it: group cardiac counseling, and group cardiac counseling combined with therapy to modify hostility, chronic rushing, and other symptoms of TABP.

His researchers studied eight hundred patients who had had a heart attack in the previous six months, dividing them into two groups, each of which would receive one or the other type of treatment. Each group met regularly for the duration of the project—four and a half years. The group in the TABP modification program learned techniques for reversing negative thinking habits, easing time urgency, relaxing the body, and altering other stress- and anger-generating behaviors. The other group received counseling without behavior modification training.

The results galvanized both the Friedman team and the cardiac community. Not only did the patients in the TABP modification program experience a greater reduction in their hostility and anger, but four and a half years after the study began, *the TABP modification patients had experienced only one quarter as many repeat heart attacks as those in the other group.*

TAKING CHARGE

More good news: you don't have to be part of a landmark study to modify your Type A characteristics. You do have to take charge of your behavior and focus your energies on changing the four main signs of the Type A behavior pattern: anxiousness, impatience, anger, and irritation, or AIAI for short.

One superb way to do this is to participate in a cardiac rehabilitation program—research has proven it. A study followed five hundred heart patients—sixty-five of whom were deemed to have highly hostile personalities—before and after they took part in rehab. The results were conclusive: rehab lowered the hostility levels and raised the quality of life of all participants but heaped the greatest benefits on the most hostile patients. Their hostility and anxiety diminished significantly, and their energy, mental health, and general well-being improved to an even greater extent than that of the less hostile patients.[15]

Another good way to control AIAI is to use my ten-step anger management program. Here it is.

ANGER MANAGEMENT, STEP 1: LAY THE FOUNDATION.

The foundation of my anger management program is anchored by two ideas—one is a truth you must accept, the other a myth you must reject:

- **You must accept that managing your anger is a critical part of your recovery from heart disease.** This has been proven beyond a doubt by numerous studies (many of which have been cited here), so it's rather simple: it's the truth, and the sooner you accept and act on it, the happier and healthier you'll be.
- **You must reject the myth that venting anger is good for you, because it isn't.**

Anger management experts agree that, contrary to popular belief, venting anger—expressing your anger in an aggressive way—does not dispel it. Rather, lashing out actually stokes your anger, working as a kind of kindling that primes you to explode at ever-smaller irritations.[16] Plus, when you vent, your aggressive behavior is highly likely to inspire the target of your tirade to respond aggressively.

What about venting when no one is around? Here, too, I advise caution. Pounding on pillows and screaming at the object of your wrath in private can indeed calm you momentarily, probably because of the relaxation that comes after you've charged yourself with adrenaline. But this kind of venting often serves as a rehearsal for inappropriate anger reactions. The next time that person irritates you, you're likely to act just as you did when you were pounding the pillow.[17]

Plus, the more you practice being angry, the better you become at it. Some cardiac researchers believe that very hostile people are prone to developing an anger habit; that is, they fly into rages over even minor annoyances because their bodies become addicted to the chemical norepinephrine, also known as noradrenaline, which the adrenal gland secretes in times of sudden stress.

Think of a bout of anger as an intense stress reaction that puts you in double jeopardy: if you express the anger in an uncontrolled way, you risk damaging your heart and your relationship with the person with whom you're annoyed. But if you repress the anger and allow it to simmer in your breast, your body responds like a car when you floor the accelerator with one foot while jamming on the brakes with the other: it goes nowhere while grinding its gears down to nubs.

To escape double jeopardy, you've got to see anger not as a fiery, uncontrollable, out-of-the-blue detonation, but as a sequence of emotions, attitudes, and behaviors that you can, with practice, learn to disrupt and defuse. A typical anger sequence unfolds like this:

1. Event
   ↓

2. Physical arousal
   ↓

3. Angry thoughts
   ↓

4. Emotional arousal
   ↓

5. Sarcasm or other critical behavior
   ↓

6. Further emotional and physical arousal
   ↓

7. Further angry thoughts

   ↓

8. Increased tension

   ↓

9. Aggressive behavior

   ↓

10. Withdrawal from others

    ↓

11. Thoughts that fuel further resentment and physical arousal

    ↓

12. Reengagement with irritable, abrupt tones

    ↓

13. Defensiveness

    ↓

14. Combativeness

    ↓

15. Disengagement.

How does this translate into real life? Well, imagine you're standing in your living room with your wife or husband—your life partner, let's say—and four bulging suitcases, waiting for your daughter (or some other do-gooder) to come and drive you to the airport. She's already fifteen minutes late, which is typical of her, and you're becoming anxious about missing your flight. Here's how things might go, according to the anger sequence detailed above:

1. Your daughter is late.

   ↓

2. Your heart rate is up; you've started to perspire.

   ↓

3. You think, "She's late, as usual. After all I've been through, you'd think she'd leave early enough to get here on time."

   ↓

4. You feel more and more angry, anxious, and restless as you repeatedly glance at your watch, noting just how late she is.

Your daughter arrives. The sequence continues.

5. You greet her with "You know, you're twenty minutes late. Are you trying to give me another heart attack?"

Your daughter responds that she hit bad traffic.

6. You've heard this a hundred times; you get more annoyed; your heart and your breathing speed up.

7. You think, "She's thirty years old, and she still can't get here on time!"

8. You glare at each other.

9. You point to the clock and shout, "Our flight leaves in less than three hours! How are we going to get there in time?"

10. You turn on your heel and march to the bathroom.

11. In the bathroom, you think of all the times your daughter has kept you waiting, and you get more and more irate.

12. You stride back into the living room and confront her: "The least you could do is start loading our suitcases in the car! Why are you just standing there?"

13. You suddenly feel self-conscious about ordering a young woman to handle your luggage: "You know I can't lift these bags myself anymore!"

Your daughter starts loading the car, muttering to herself and straining to lift the suitcases.

14. Now you're really a mess—ashamed and angry, you assert your authority: "Be careful with my carry-on—it's got all my medicine in it!"

15. Finally the car is loaded. Your daughter starts the engine. Your spouse, who hasn't said a word, sits stonily in the front seat. You crawl into the back and don't speak for the rest of the drive.

When you're dancing on emotional land mines, explosions seem inevitable. But they aren't. What we typically refer to as anger actually involves three distinct phenomena: emotion (the anger itself); thoughts (the attitudes and beliefs you hold which feed your anger); and behaviors (the actions you take to express your anger).

ANGER MANAGEMENT, STEP 2:
LEARN THE DIFFERENCE BETWEEN ANGER AND AROUSAL.

The second step in my anger management program is articulated by the authors of an excellent book entitled *When Anger Hurts,*[18] who remind us that the body responds similarly when we feel rushed, frustrated, annoyed, sexually aroused, frightened, embarrassed, challenged, excited, or angry. (In other words, if your heart is pounding and your palms are moist, you might not be angry; you might be in love, or late for an appointment, or surprised to see your ex-sweetheart in the arms of someone you work with.) With practice, you can learn to figure out what you're feeling and use the information to interrupt anger reactions. A good way to start is by keeping an anger journal. Get a small notebook, a stack of index cards, or a memo pad. Write today's date at the top of the first page and start keeping track of your moods:

- Periodically throughout the day—say, every two hours—note the number of times you got angry since your last entry.
- Next, rate how aroused you felt during those moments of anger. Try to differentiate *physical arousal*—signs of the fight-or-flight syndrome such as rapid heart rate, shallow breathing, muscular tension, and so on— from *emotional arousal*—how angry you felt. Use a scale of one to ten, with one indicating minimal arousal or anger and ten indicating intense arousal or anger.

Keeping an anger journal will help you in several ways. First, it is important to recognize when your behavior misrepresents what you are feeling. Those around you may mistake your expressions of emotional arousal for those of anger. But if your journal entries suggest that you are indeed getting angry several times a day, analyze your situation and create an action plan. Start by noting what stirred your anger. If the cause isn't clear to you, note what may have stressed you before the angry episode. Ask yourself, *What was I feeling before I got angry? Am I blocking a feeling or source of stress by being angry?* You may figure out that the reason you snapped at the coffee wagon attendant was because she was the first person you saw after you called home four times and kept getting a busy signal.

Also, take time to analyze your journal entries. Read through them each night and ask yourself:

- What sorts of people and situations tend to make me angry?
- What work situations make me angry, and why?
- How do I usually respond to my own anger and the anger of others? Do I overreact, give in, blame others, repress my feelings, or express them inappropriately?
- What feelings are lurking behind the angry ones? Do I get angry when I feel rejected, ashamed, unworthy, afraid?

ANGER MANAGEMENT, STEP 3:
LEARN WHAT YOUR ANGER IS ABOUT.

I have never counseled a heart patient who could gain control of his or her anger and hostility without grasping this truth: other people may stir your feelings, but **your anger is *your* anger; it is intimately entwined with what is inside you, and you must learn to take responsibility for it.** In *Anger: Wisdom for Cooling the Flames,* Buddhist master Thich Nhat Hanh recommends thinking of anger as a seed within you.[19] This anger seed holds the emotional residue of your history and psychology. Some situations and people may fertilize the seed and cause it to germinate, but your anger is embedded in your personal dealings with yourself, and you must disengage it by the roots from the dark soil of the self.

In many years of counseling heart patients, I have learned that unresolved grief often bleeds beneath the skin of chronic anger and hostility. As mentioned earlier, the disappointments and losses that come with heart illness can beset a person with grief, and anger is a stage of the grieving process. As you contemplate what your anger is about, ask yourself: *What losses have been particularly difficult for me to bear, and how am I coping with them?*

Clément, a forty-nine-year-old actor living in Los Angeles, walked around with jaw pain for three weeks until one afternoon it seized him with such force he asked his wife, Marguerite, to take him to the local clinic. Tall, dark, lanky, and handsome, Clément didn't look like someone with heart trouble. But when he collapsed in the examining room, he was rushed to the hospital for an emergency angioplasty. Here is what Clément said about the anger he felt at being diagnosed with heart disease:

> *"The whole episode paled in comparison to having to quit cigarettes. At my fol-low-up visit to the cardiologist after being released from the hospital, I was a basket case. And I lit into him—I felt bad about it later—I told him, 'You know, this heart thing was a nonevent in my life in comparison to having to quit cigarettes.' And I was deep in the throes of withdrawal for a week to ten days after that.*
>
> *"I felt a tremendous amount of resentment. It makes no sense emotionally; this was the guy who pretty much saved my life, or at least saved me from severe heart damage. But he was the one who was most immediately insistent, saying, 'That's it—you'll never touch a cigarette again.'*
>
> *"For me, it felt like a fifth limb had been severed. I'd been smoking about three quarters of a pack a day since I was fifteen; about thirty-five years. It becomes a part of your life—when you're talking on the phone, after a meal, when you take ten during rehearsal, during intermission . . . smoking was my friend, in good times, bad times, indifferent times, the cigarette was always there.*
>
> *"People would ask, 'How're you feeling? How're you feeling?,' and you really want to say, 'Will you stop?' It's supportive and caring, but for the one on the receiving end, there's the unspoken question, which is 'Are you still off ciga-rettes?' You really want to say, 'Mind your own damn business. Let's talk about something else.' "*

In Clément's case, rage at having to give up cigarettes was a manifestation of grief. His decision to choose life and quit smoking in no way diminished the grief he felt at losing the habit. He had to face this loss and endure the pain before he could start to feel better.

If your anger flows from unfinished grieving, you too must face your loss and feel the pain before you can heal. This means finding someone you trust to whom you can talk about what you're feeling. Talking to a trusted friend, family member, therapist, or spiritual leader about painful emotions and accepting his or her support will not only ease your suffering but also avert physical health complications that can arise when these feelings are suppressed.

Let yourself fully feel and talk about your losses. You might find it help-ful to write about your feelings, expressing what you cherished and regret-ted about the friendship, person, or situation that you lost. Remember: Grieving is a process that diminishes in intensity when you experience it fully. Let others be of help to you and be patient with yourself. With the comfort of friends and compassion toward yourself, you can grieve in safety until you are relieved.

Anger Management, Step 4: Calm Down.

If you have an anger habit, it means your calming response isn't kicking in on its own and you must deliberately calm down. You do this by learning to recognize the signs that your fuse has been lit and stamping it out before you explode.

You can disarm an anger sequence by interrupting it. Deliberately will yourself to thrust a moment of relaxation, humor, affection, compassion, inquisitiveness, or spiritual communion into the midst of your anger buildup. This means doing any of a number of things you've probably done unconsciously from time to time but never thought about doing deliberately. Acting deliberately to calm angry impulses prompts the brain to release endorphins, chemicals that inhibit pain and derail violent physical reactions.

EXERCISE OR MEDICATION—OR BOTH—MIGHT HELP

As few as three months of regular aerobic exercise yields critical physical changes that can help you manage your anger. First, by exposing your body to physical stress when you exercise, you'll lower the amount of physical arousal you experience when you're emotionally stressed, making it less likely that you'll fly off the handle and also reducing distress to your cardiovascular system.[20]

Recent research also suggests that the SSRI antidepressant medications discussed in Chapter 7 may also help curb chronic hostile reactions.[21] When you pair an SSRI with the self-help strategies described in this chapter, you can profoundly change your anger reactions.

Anger Management, Step 5: Control Anger-Generating Thoughts.

Getting angry seems to go fist-in-fist with anger-provoking thinking. Psychologist Robert Allan emphasizes that you fuel your anger when you convince yourself that someone is either doing you an injustice or intentionally behaving in an incompetent way.[22] Anger expert Henri Weisenger points out that we indulge in anger-generating thoughts not only when others disappoint us, but when we fall short of the expectations we have of ourselves—which are often inflated, if not grandiose.[23]

Countering Angry Thoughts

One way to counter angry thoughts is to practice empathy, the virtue of being able to put yourself in another person's place and view him or her with compassion, if not approval. When you're angry, remind yourself that others are usually doing their best—however mediocre it may be—given who they are and what their lives have taught them; that everyone moves at his or her own pace (which is sometimes much slower than yours); and that no one set out in the morning with the mission to infuriate you.

This isn't always easy to do. When patients ask me how they can develop empathy, I suggest they use coping statements. Coping statements are tools you can use to counter anger. The idea is to use them to talk back to your anger-provoking self-talk. The next time you find yourself starting to seethe, arrest your angry thoughts and replace them with one or more of the coping statements I've printed below. If they don't sound enough like you to feel natural, change the words until you can imagine yourself using them. If you feel awkward directing your thinking by using words, try to get over your prejudice. It may feel forced at first, but remember: you're retraining your reactions, and reacting to others with empathy rather than rage can save your life.

COPING STATEMENTS

- "I can't accomplish anything by blaming other people, even if they are responsible for the problem. I'll try another angle."
- "I may not like it, but she (or he) is probably doing her best right now."
- "I have a choice about how to react right now. I will choose wisely."
- "Will this matter five years from now? (Five hours? Five minutes?)"
- "If I'm still angry about this tomorrow, I'll deal with it then. But for now I'm just going to cool off."
- "I'm free to want what I want, but he (or she) is free to want something else."
- "I'm not in charge of the world, nor of the people in it. It's not my job to make everything right."

- "Getting angry will not get me what I want."
- "Acting angry is not the same as showing that I care."
- "Calmness is not a weakness; it is a sign of power."
- "Let me ask rather than tell."
- "I'll listen rather than talk."
- "This is maddening but it's also interesting. Let me try to figure it out."
- "Remember to laugh."
- "I'm in charge of how I react; they aren't."
- "I deserve to enjoy my life. I won't allow anyone to deprive me of that pleasure."
- "Hostility is hazardous to my health."
- "It takes strength and maturity to show love and compassion."
- "The fastest way is not necessarily the best way except in a life-or-death situation, and this is not one of them."
- "How big is this issue, compared to the size of my life?"

Anger Management, Step 6: Decide Whether You Must Take Action or if It Just Feels That Way.

When you're really angry and vibrating with an adrenaline rush, you're primed to take action—any action—no matter how wrong-headed it is and how much you may regret it later. If you're a person whose hostility frequently catapults you into the vibration zone, you're probably reacting in ways that are as destructive to your heart and relationships as they are unnecessary.

Psychiatrist Redford Williams is one of the pioneers of behavioral medicine and credited with spearheading the research that forged the link between hostility and heart illness. In *Anger Kills,* he and coauthor Virginia Williams offer a simple template for controlling angry reactions: stop, regain control of yourself, ask yourself the following questions, and let the answers dictate what you do next: [24]

1. Would a jury of impartial observers decide that this situation warrants my being angry?
2. If the jury agrees that your anger is justified, ask yourself:
   a. Is this a situation I must remedy?
   b. Is it worth the effort I would have to expend to remedy the situation?
   c. If so, is there something I can actually *do* to remedy the situation?

If the answer to any of these questions is no, then switch to a self-soothing strategy. Ask yourself, "What would help me let this situation go?"

If you decide you do want to take action and that doing so will improve a situation that is important to you, then you must decide what, specifically, would help. Ask yourself, "To whom may I speak, and what should I say? What can I do? What should I do?"

As you prepare to take action, keep in mind that you do not have to be angry to rectify a wrong. In fact, because anger is an altered state of consciousness in which you think neither quickly nor clearly, you should marshal all your powers to resist the urge to lash out. Wait until you cool off a bit; then deal with the conflict. But by a bit, I mean a bit, not a month. Don't wait until the situation is cold, old news. A good guideline is to discuss what is bothering you before you become irate—while the iron is still warming up—or within twenty-four hours of the anger episode—while the iron is cooling off. And remember to be assertive, not aggressive. The objective is to ease a thorny situation, not create a new one.

ANGER MANAGEMENT, STEP 7: CONTROL YOUR BEHAVIORS.

The next step in managing anger is not psychological, it's behavioral; it's not about changing how you think but how you act. Even if you have trouble controlling angry thoughts and feelings, you can safeguard your heart health, your marriage or primary partnership, and all your relationships if you control the urge to act aggressively.

Controlling yourself is not only tactful, it's wise. Changing the way you express yourself when you're in conflict—for example, dismantling verbal bombs and using less explosive language—lowers the strain on your heart even if you are extremely angry, frustrated, or both.[25]

To modify the way you express yourself, start paying attention to these six aspects of your communication style, especially when you're angry:[26]

1. **The words you use:** Do you use curse words, insults, or sarcasm when your temper flares?

2. **The sounds you make:** Do you sigh irritably or use other vocalizations to convey your annoyance?

3. **The quality, tone, and volume of your voice:** Does your voice take on an edge when you're upset? Do you speak more loudly or more softly than when you're relaxed?

4. **Your hand and arm gestures:** Do you ever shake your fist in a menacing way or point your finger in the face of someone who's annoying you?

5. **Your facial expressions:** Do you exaggerate your facial expressions to convey your hostility?

6. **Your body movements:** Do you move your body differently when you're angry?

At the first prickles of irritation, reprogram your habitual anger behaviors by remembering to:

- Focus on one problem at a time.
- Decide what the problem actually is.
- Express your feelings honestly, but not belligerently.
- Avoid belittling or otherwise insulting the object of your wrath.
- Separate the person from the problem.
- Be gracious and give the person you're in conflict with the benefit of the doubt.
- Ask the person to help you resolve the problem, even if he or she created it.
- Avoid making judgments about the other person's character.
- Resist the temptation to bully or threaten the person with whom you're in conflict.
- Use "I" statements to express what you think, feel, need, or want, as opposed to "you" statements, which express your opinion of the other person.
- Suggest ways to remedy the problem rather than decry the problem's existence.
- State that you hope to move beyond the tension and toward conciliation.
- Preserve your self-respect, and refrain from attempting to damage that of the other person.
- Thank the other person for taking time to work through the problem with you.

My patients also find it useful to learn from politicians and be equipped with a few prepared statements when they're not confident they can express themselves eloquently. Memorizing responses before you need them isn't phony; rather, it's a way to ensure your ability to speak in a reasonable way when your reason has already fled the premises. I recommend my patients choose from among the following five phrases, which I've adapted from *When Anger Hurts:*

1. I'm feeling _____ , and what I think I need (*or* want *or* would like) is _____ .
2. What would you propose we do to solve this problem?
3. If this situation continues, I'll have to _____ to take care of myself.
4. What do you need in this situation? *Or,* What concerns (or bothers) you about this situation?
5. So, if I understand correctly, what you want is _____ .

Before you decide these sentences sound too unnatural or corny to be useful, try to imagine using them. Let's say you've just learned that your significant other has invited two couples you're friendly with to dinner. The invitation was proffered with the hope that it would cheer and distract you; however, you feel a rush of anxiety and annoyance about having to entertain guests that evening. Rather than lash out, you could use a rehearsed response—in this case, number 1 or 5 above—to express your dismay without worsening the situation:

1. "I'm feeling anxious at the thought of having company—I don't think I'm ready. I'd feel better if we waited a little longer before having people over."
5. "I understand you want to cheer me up, and you thought that seeing my friends would do the trick. I love you for that. But I don't think I'm ready, and would appreciate it if you'd call them and reschedule for a later date."

As with the coping statements I offered earlier, adapt the vocabulary and cadence of these responses to sound like you. It's not the wording but the essence of the statement that matters.

ANGER MANAGEMENT, STEP 8: DON'T GET HOOKED.

A hook is an unexpected, inconsequential irritant or stressor with the potential to rile you well beyond its true significance. It's unexpected because it's suddenly dangling in front of your nose, and it's inconsequential in the grand scheme of things, but if you swallow it, it could tear you up plenty before you're able to free yourself. Hooks come in myriad forms: the receptionist who puts you on hold without saying hello; the maître d' who gives away your table when you're in the bathroom; the kid who demands for the eighty-fifth time that you buy him hundred-dollar sneakers; or the coworker who asks you yet again if you can cover the phones for her while she steps away from her desk. None of these situations merits a heated verbal assault, but you could easily launch one if you swallow the hook. It's been estimated that the average urban worker encounters thirty-two hooks a day!

The hook metaphor was created by Lynda Powell, Ph.D., a researcher who studies Type A behaviors and ways of modifying them.[27] She suggests that people visualize potential stressors as hooks they can choose to either swim past or swallow. When a hook suddenly floats into view, don't bite. Instead, ask yourself the following questions:

- Am I going to let this person or situation manipulate my feelings?
- Why should I punish myself for others' mistakes by getting upset and harming my health?
- Am I going to waste my precious time letting this situation agitate me or will I use my time to find a way to make things better?

The key here is, of course, to learn to discern between situations that warrant spirited emotional reactions and those that don't. Think of yourself as a highly intelligent and disciplined fish: if you keep your mouth shut, you won't get hooked.

Anger Management, Step 9:
When Things Heat Up, Call a Time-Out.

Calling a time-out—stepping back from a contentious situation, taking some deep breaths, and calming yourself before rejoining the fray—is an effective way to disrupt an anger sequence. Disengaging yourself from a confrontation allows you to calm your body, collect your thoughts, and take a more constructive approach with whomever or whatever is bothering you.

But calling a time-out works only if you use it appropriately. Don't use the break to fuel your anger by replaying the conflict in your mind, revving up your body, or both. Don't duck into a restaurant and order a cappuccino, a cola, or a glass of chardonnay; caffeine will only make your heart beat faster and sustain your agitation, and alcohol will make it harder to control your emotions and your tongue when you return to the conversation. During a time-out, it's wise to avoid both stimulants and depressants, whether food, beverages, or drugs. You should also avoid potentially stressful activities such as driving or getting drawn into a competitive video game.

Instead, use the time to relieve tension in a healthy way. Release angry thoughts; try to relax and clear your mind. Attempt to see the problem from your antagonist's perspective, not because he or she is right but because it may grant you insight into how to deal with the person in terms that he or she can accept. Remember: if you are able to feel compassion, your anger will diminish.

After a suitable time—I recommend at least thirty minutes—take charge and reopen the conversation. If you are still unable to conduct yourself with compassion and control, request an appointment to resolve the conflict at a later date or time.

ANGER MANAGEMENT, STEP 10: SLOW DOWN.

Slowing down is one of the most effective ways to gain control of your emotions and your life. If you're one of those people who is convinced you'll run out of time unless you operate at warp speed, do yourself and the people around you a favor by slowing down.

Speak more slowly, and resist the temptation to interrupt others. This will calm you and provide you with a feeling of control (over yourself, if no one else). People will enjoy your company more if you allow them to finish their own sentences.

Here are more tips for countering hurry sickness, courtesy of the redoubtable Dr. Friedman and the Recurrent Coronary Prevention Project: [28]

- Ask yourself at least once a week: "What is causing me to rush so much? What is inspiring my exaggerated sense of urgency?"
- Remind yourself each morning that life is, by its very nature, unfinished, and that you should not expect all your projects to neatly conclude at a chosen (and usually arbitrary) time.
- Stop thinking about and doing more than one thing at a time.
- Do not interfere when someone is doing a job more slowly than you could.
- Whenever you can, use your money to buy time. Pay someone to mow the lawn, iron your shirts, clean the house, and do other time-consuming chores that compound your compulsion to rush.
- Don't assume that others are as concerned about time as you are.
- Interrupt lengthy work sessions with relaxation breaks.
- Appreciate beauty wherever and in whatever form you find it.

- Resist the urge to drive in the fast lane. Also, try to stay in the same lane, without weaving in and out to pass drivers who are crawling along at sixty-five miles an hour.

- Establish calming rituals in your daily life: sit down at breakfast to read the newspaper, do a crossword puzzle at lunchtime, learn to knit or crochet, read before bed, take up meditation.

- Walk, talk, and eat more slowly.

- Spend ten minutes each evening recalling the day's events.

- Do nothing but listen to soothing music for fifteen minutes.

- Ask a member of your family about his or her day and—here's the challenge—*listen* to the answer.

- Ask yourself: "What did I do right today, and what happened that is worth remembering?"

- Periodically hear out another person—no matter how long-winded he or she is—without interrupting even once.

It really all comes down to an old-fashioned practice that I recommend to all my patients: practice patience.

Chapter Nine

RECLAIM YOUR SEX LIFE AND PHYSICAL INTIMACY

(But You'll Have to Get Off the Couch)

Here's a quiz:

In the first six months after a heart attack, what do four out of five people say they are afraid to do?

(a) Return to work.

(b) Visit their in-laws.

(c) Have sex.

(d) Watch one of those shows about how they do a face-lift.

If you picked (d), alas, you are incorrect: 100 percent of all people, whether or not they've had a heart attack, are afraid to watch a face-lift. No, the correct answer is (c): four out of five people say they are afraid to have sex for six months after a heart attack. Partners of heart patients also worry, afraid to make love now that heart disease has invaded their bedrooms.

But while sexual anxiety among heart patients and their partners is common, it also passes: 40 to 75 percent of heart patients who were sexually active at the time of their diagnosis *do* return to having sexual relations, albeit with modifications in some cases.[1] Definitive statistics are unavailable because estimates vary among studies and variations of the disease; nonetheless, here is some of what we know:

- **Myocardial infarction (MI, or heart attack).** After suffering a myocardial infarction, about a quarter of patients stop having sex, another quarter report no change in their sex lives, and half report that they continue to enjoy sex, but less frequently than before.[2]

- **Coronary artery bypass graft (CABG) and percutaneous transluminal coronary angioplasty (PTCA).** While CABG, commonly known as a bypass, has more immediate sexual effects than PTCA, known as angioplasty, the sexual effects of the procedures even out within fifteen months of surgery. A survey of CABG patients found that, slightly sooner than eight weeks after the bypass, 47 percent were making love as often as before, 36 percent were doing it less often, and 8 percent weren't doing it at all. On an encouraging note, nearly 10 percent of CABG patients said they were making love *more often* than before the surgery.[3]

- **Heart failure (HF).** In a study of fifty-one men and eleven women with advanced heart failure, approximately three-quarters of them reported a marked decrease in sexual interest and frequency of sexual relations, and one-quarter ceased sexual activity altogether. Half the patients, men and women alike, said the pleasure or satisfaction they normally derived from sex dropped significantly once heart failure developed.[4] The effects of advanced heart failure are clear: in the later stages of this illness, most patients report either little or no interest in sex and consequently seldom engage in it. (For more on HF, see Chapter 11.)

- **Pacemaker.** Nearly seven of ten pacemaker recipients younger than sixty-five say their sex lives haven't changed as a result of having the device. The remaining 30 percent are evenly divided between reporting their sex lives have gotten either better or worse.[5]

- **Automatic implantable cardiodefibrillator (ICD).** Six out of ten ICD patients say their sex lives didn't change after receiving the device, while four out of ten say their sex lives changed for the worse. (For details on living with an ICD, see Chapter 12.)

- **Heart transplant.** Most transplant recipients are sexually inactive before the surgery. In a study of men who were sexually active before their transplants, nearly half reported no change in their sex lives after the transplant; 29 percent said their sex lives improved, and 23 percent said their sex lives got worse.[6]

- **Heart pump, or left ventricular assist device (LVAD).** As I write this, there is news that heart pumps, currently used to keep transplant candidates alive while they await donor hearts, may soon be approved as permanent implants for people with severe congestive heart failure.[7] At this time there is insufficient information about the effect of LVADs on sexual activity.

- **Peripheral arterial disease (PAD).** PAD is diagnosed when a patient's circulation is impaired and not enough blood reaches the extremities. Primary symptoms of PAD include cramping in muscles of the buttocks, thighs, or calves, especially when the patient is at rest. About half of PAD patients suffer from impaired sexual response, its most common manifestation in men being difficulty achieving or sustaining an erection.[8]

The salient point is this: **Sex after heart illness isn't dangerous, but it isn't simple, either.** When you have heart disease, new and confounding factors climb into bed with you that make sex a more complex undertaking than it was before. Anxiety, self-consciousness, aging, and medication side effects can bedevil even the lustiest partnership. And that's where the complexity comes in: it's not always heart illness that's the problem, at least not the only problem. Many people blame their sexual difficulties on heart illness (or the medications they take for it) when the sex problem actually came first. Patients assume their difficulties are a result of emotional upheaval; then, when things calm down, they don't understand why their intimacy problems persist. There are many reasons: diabetes, depression, clogged arteries, high blood pressure, and just plain aging are just a few conditions that affect sexual arousal, and no one escapes them all.

That said, the vast majority of heart patients who enjoyed sex before their illness enjoy sex again afterward. Many of my patients say the increased closeness and affection they have developed with their partners because of the illness has improved their sex lives. This renewal of intimacy typically begins when patients and their partners decide to face rather than avoid their problems, however awkward it may feel to do so.

TYPES OF SEXUAL PROBLEMS

Sexual performance problems include reduction or lack of desire (low sex drive), difficulty becoming aroused or erect (these include female arousal disorder and male erectile dysfunction), and disorders of orgasm and ejaculation. In 1999, *The American Journal of Cardiology* noted with dismay that sexual dysfunction among women has been sorely neglected and denounced the lack of counseling and information available to female heart patients compared to that available to males.[9] This is an appalling oversight, given the fact that sexual dysfunction is more common in females than in males overall, affecting 20 to 50 percent of American women.[10] If you're a woman with heart illness and are having sexual difficulties, you must make a point of getting help. Chances are slim that any of your doctors will ask you about your sex life unless you bring it up. If you think you're too shy to discuss it, practice talking about it at home before you visit your doctor so the words will seem less charged when you need to speak them. Sexuality is a fundamental part of life and a significant aspect of your health; you owe it to yourself to face the problem and get help.

With men, erectile dysfunction (ED) is the most frequently diagnosed and treated sexual problem. Men who have heart disease are more likely to suffer from ED than those who don't[11]—50 to 75 percent of men experience some sexual dysfunction after a heart attack. But it's also true that many of these men had sexual problems before they had heart problems.[12] The Massachusetts Male Aging Study, which surveyed 1290 men living in eleven randomly selected towns near Boston between 1987 and 1989, reported that over half of those who were between the ages of forty and seventy had some degree of ED from time to time, and that the prevalence increased with age, reaching 70 percent when the men reached seventy years of age.[13]

You'd think that erectile dysfunction is something that all physicians would discuss with their male patients, especially those with heart disease but, strangely enough, it isn't: *six out of ten male heart patients say they received no sex counseling over the course of their recovery.*[14] That's what Frank said when he came to my office. A tanned and muscular fifty-two-year-old construction worker, Frank finally got around to broaching the subject after thirty minutes of small talk:

"Like I said, I'm feeling okay, but I'm worried about one thing . . . let's just say that my bedroom behavior has changed since the heart attack, and I'm not talking about sleeping.

"When things get going, the first thing I notice is my heartbeat—it fills up my head. My breathing gets faster, too. And as I get more into it, I feel my heart pounding in my chest. That's when I get scared—I start worrying, am I going to have another heart attack? I get obsessed with it, and I can't stop. It's all I can think about."

(There was in fact another explanation for Frank's rapid breathing and pounding heart: he was turned on and about to have sex.)

THE GREAT NEWS: YOU *WILL* HAVE SEX AGAIN

It is perfectly normal for recently diagnosed heart patients to worry that physical exertion of any sort—including sex—might trigger another cardiac event. I have treated hundreds of patients like Frank who, because no one talked to them about it, confused the signs of normal sexual arousal with symptoms of a heart attack. Both inside and outside the bedroom (or wherever you prefer to make love), you'll reclaim confidence that you can conduct a normal life, including a sexual one, when you have experience living your new normal, when you know the facts, and when you've learned how to cope with your concerns.

FIRST, THE FACTS

The truth about sex and heart disease is shrouded in myth, spun from yarns such as: "I knew a guy who had a cousin whose brother-in-law went, *wham!*—just like that!—died of a heart attack in the sack," and so on. Such tales breed fear and offer little insight about sex and the heart. Yes, some people *do* die while they're having sex. Others die while grocery shopping, watching television, sleeping, or taking out the trash. That doesn't mean that any of these activities is inherently dangerous, or that we're about to stop doing them.

Cardiologist James E. Muller and his colleagues at Massachusetts General Hospital recently conducted a study that has become the last word on heart attack triggers, in both healthy people and heart patients.[15] Muller's team interviewed more than 1,700 men and women a week after they suffered a myocardial infarction (MI). Citing a statistic noted earlier—that a healthy fifty-year-old man who exercises regularly has only a one-in-a-million per hour chance of having an MI[16]—the team concluded that sexual activity provoked an MI in fewer than seventeen of the cases—that's less than 1 percent. Specifically, for two hours after having sex, the risk of heart attack for healthy men and women rose from one in a million to only 2.5 in a million. For heart attack survivors, the risk rose to *only 2.9 in a million*— barely more than that for healthy folks.

As for other triggers, studies have reported that a burst of anger increases the risk of MI to 2.3 in a million,[17] and vigorous physical exertion raises the risk to 5.9 in a million.[18] This means that, in most cases, the chances of having a heart attack after sex are no greater than those of having one after an argument and considerably less than those of having one after carrying a piano up four flights of stairs.[19] And if you've had a bypass or angioplasty there's more good news: as long as you're not currently suffering from angina, your risk of having a heart attack during sex is no greater than that of a heart patient who hasn't had the surgery.[20]

As for the type of sexual activity, that's not an issue, either . . . for the most part. First, the cardiac demands of sexual intercourse are only slightly greater than those of arousal from either self-stimulation or partner stimulation. And regarding the missionary position, there seems to be little difference in cardiac strain between man-on-top and woman-on-top variations.

But what about an extraordinary sexual encounter, one that's wildly, thrillingly *different?* Some people believe that the potential danger of sex is affected by three Ps: place, partner, and position. They think that having sex in an exotic setting or with a new partner (especially one with whom you shouldn't be cavorting in the first place) or in an unfamiliar position may increase cardiac strain and lead to a heart attack. As tempting as it is to use this to intimidate folks into behaving themselves, there's no reputable research to support the notion that novel, ravishing sex is any more dangerous than the same-old, same-old kind. And barring acrobatics à la Cirque du Soleil, one position seems to be as safe as another.

Far more perilous than making love on the couch is sitting there for hours, potatolike, in front of the TV. The biggest favor you can do yourself is to get into shape, because the fitter you are, the lower your chances of having a cardiac event during sex. For sedentary people with heart illness, the risk that sudden heavy exertion will cause an MI *approaches one in 1,000—a thousand times greater* than the one-in-a-million odds for healthy, active males.[21] In the Muller study, *only two heart attacks occurred in people accustomed to regular, vigorous exercise* (the kind that reddens your face and makes you pant).

HOW RED MUST YOU GET?

That all depends on what you want to accomplish.

Cardiac rehabilitation specialists use three main factors to gauge the heart's capacity to tolerate exertion and excitement: oxygen consumption, heart rate, and blood pressure. Oxygen consumption is measured by calculating its metabolic equivalent, known as a MET level. Your MET level is a general indicator of your overall cardiac fitness; it provides a measurement of your heart's ability to keep up with the body's varying oxygen demands. MET levels are calculated according to the oxygen requirement of an activity rather than its duration; whether you wash windows for five minutes or forty-five, the activity requires 4.5 METs. (However, if you're washing windows like a lunatic five minutes before your company arrives, that could crank you up to 6 to 7 METs.) MET levels have been assigned to various activities, including the following.[22]

ACTIVITY	METS
Sleeping	.9
Sitting quietly (riding in a car, listening to music, watching TV)	1
Sitting and knitting or sewing	1.5
Sitting in class or at a meeting	1.8
Ironing	2.3

Cooking and preparing food	2.5
Cleaning, light (dusting, vacuuming, changing linens)	2.5
Cleaning, heavy (washing car or windows; cleaning garage)	4.5
Mowing lawn, power mower	4.5
Mowing lawn, manual (push) mower	6
Golf, using power cart	3.5
Golf, pulling clubs	5
Golf, carrying clubs	5.5
Walking at 2 mph, level, firm surface	2.5
Walking for pleasure, work break, walking the dog	3.5
Walking at 3.5 mph, level, firm surface	4
Walking at 3.5 mph, uphill	6
Walking, downstairs	3
Walking, upstairs	8
Stretching, hatha yoga	4
Swimming—backstroke	8
Swimming—breaststroke	10
Swimming—crawl	11
Dancing—fast (folk, disco, square)	5.5
Dancing—slow (waltz, fox-trot)	3
Bicycling, leisure (<10 mph)	4
Bicycling, leisure (10–12 mph)	6
Bicycling, leisure (12–14 mph)	8
Bicycling, leisure (14–16 mph)	10
Farming, milking by hand	3
Shopping for milk at market	3.5

Clearly, if you're an avid exerciser, you have nothing to worry about. But even if you're not, you should be fine: **Within several weeks of suffering an MI, most patients have a 6-to-9-MET capacity.** Which, as you'll see from the chart that follows, is more than you need:

ACTIVITY	METS
Preorgasmic arousal: sexual play	2–3 [23]
Sexual intercourse	2.5–3.3 on average, depending on position [24]
Orgasm	3–4 [25]

Of course, MET levels for sex vary somewhat according to what you do, how long you do it, and your general level of comfort while doing it. Generally, the upper range of cardiac exertion during sex requires about 5 to 6 METs in younger people and less in older people (as well as those in a long-established relationship).

Research into heart rate is also encouraging. In a classic study conducted by Drs. Herman Hellerstein and E. H. Friedman,[26] ninety-one young cardiac rehab patients—average age forty-seven—wore portable electrocardiograph monitors for two days and nights while going about their normal routines. For fourteen male patients, the normal routines included sex. According to the mini-EKGs, at the moment of climax, the patients' heart rates ranged from 90 to 144 beats per minute, with an average of 117—*lower than the 120 average beats per minute recorded as patients went through their daily routines!* (A more recent study reported heart rate increases of 50 to 60 beats per minute over baseline, up to 130 beats per minute, during sex.[27])

As for blood pressure, you shouldn't worry about that either (unless you have high blood pressure, in which case worry is warranted—see p. 164). Hellerstein and Friedman's study estimated mean blood pressure during intercourse at a modest 162 systolic/89 diastolic; according to guidelines revised in 2003, normal blood pressure is 119/79, and that's *not* during sex (see box, p. 25). Moreover, in a fifteen-minute lovemaking session, the spike in blood pressure lasts for only three to five minutes.[28] And it's no different if you have heart disease: studies report these same heart rate and blood pressure figures for both heart attack survivors and patients with stable angina.

If you're taking cardiac medication, you may have even lower heart rate and pressure readings, as some medications lower heart strain during sex. One study of angina patients noted that without medication, participants' heart rates during sexual intercourse averaged 122 beats per minute but dropped to 82 if they were taking a beta-blocker drug. (Beta-blockers are a class of medications commonly prescribed to treat angina. They lower heart rate by hindering the effects of adrenaline [epinephrine] and noradrenaline [norepinephrine] on the heart.) The beta-blockade relieved angina symptoms in 65 percent of patients who reported angina-related pain during sex.[29]

THE NOT-SO-GREAT NEWS

I do have some words of caution about sex and heart illness. First, some people do experience irregular heartbeats during sex, probably because the sympathetic nervous system becomes activated by the emotions that sexual activity often involves. This can lead to ventricular tachycardia, a heart rhythm disturbance characterized by a very rapid heartbeat that can lead to further complications.

Second, a serious warning to those who enjoy anal intercourse or stimulation of the outer portion of the anus: insertion of *any object* into the anus can be dangerous for heart patients. Anal penetration often causes stimulation of the vagus nerve, which can send heart rate plummeting and cause dizziness or loss of consciousness. If you enjoy anal sex and have heart disease, you would be wise to focus on the erotic potential of stimulation to the anal area without penetration. In any case, you should avoid deep anal penetration.

Finally, be aware that, if you have high blood pressure (hypertension) and are not taking medication to control it, it may be dangerous for you to have an orgasm. I've counseled many patients who dutifully filled their blood pressure medication prescriptions, took the drugs for a while, then stopped taking them because the side effects dampened their sex lives. The irony is, of course, that stopping the medication may improve your sexual response, but sex without the medication could be very dangerous to your heart. A British study found that men with mild hypertension (155/87) who did not take pressure-lowering medication reached pressures of 237/138 at the moment of orgasm—well within the perilous range.[30] Again, this spike lasted an average of only three to five minutes out of a quarter-hour lovemaking session,[31] but the point stands: if you have high blood pressure and are not taking medication for it, you would do well to avoid reaching climax.

IS SEX SAFE FOR YOU? EVALUATE YOUR RISK PROFILE

In 1999, Princeton University hosted an international conference on sexual activity and cardiac risk. One of the many fruits of that conference was a set of sexual guidelines for heart patients published in *The American Journal of Cardiology* and adapted here.[32] To evaluate your own profile, start reading the following list of major risk factors for cardiovascular disease and check any that apply to you:

____ I am over sixty-five years old.

____ I am male.

____ I am a postmenopausal female.

____ I have high blood pressure.

____ I have diabetes.

____ I am obese (20 percent or more over the midpoint of your weight range on a standard height-weight table).[33]

___ I smoke cigarettes.

___ I have an elevated cholesterol level (dyslipidimia).

___ I tend to be sedentary rather than physically active.

INTERPRETING THE QUESTIONNAIRE: ARE YOU AT LOW RISK?

According to the experts, you are at **low risk** of suffering a cardiac event from sexual activity if all the following apply:

- You checked only one or two risk factors.
- You do not have high blood pressure or, if you do, you control it by taking medication.
- If you have angina, it is mild and stable (a physician has evaluated your symptoms and is treating them, if necessary).
- If you had a CABG (bypass) or PCTA intervention (angioplasty, stenting [placement in the artery of a small tube, or stent, to keep vessel open], or the like), your physician has deemed the procedure a success.
- If you have valvular disease such as mitral valve or aortic stenosis, the condition is mild.
- If you have congestive heart failure (CHF), it is class I, the mildest and typically asymptomatic form (see Chapter 11).
- If you had a heart attack, six to eight weeks have elapsed since the event. (The period of sexual inactivity can be shortened to three to four weeks in patients who have satisfactorily completed post-MI stress testing. Heart surgery patients are often ready to resume sexual relations as soon as three weeks after discharge from the hospital. Many choose to wait longer because they don't feel mentally or physically ready for sex. A cardiac event is most likely to occur within two weeks of an MI.)

If the above-described conditions resemble your own, you are probably at **low risk** of suffering cardiac complications due to sex, and special testing and evaluation should not be necessary before your physician clears you to either resume sexual relations or receive treatment for sexual problems (including medications to enhance arousal).

INTERPRETING THE QUESTIONNAIRE: ARE YOU AT MODERATE RISK?

You are at **moderate risk** of suffering a cardiac event from sexual activity if the following conditions apply to you:

- You have three or more risk factors. (Sedentary lifestyle is particularly significant because the lack of physical conditioning increases the cardiac risk of sexual activity as well as other forms of physical exertion.)
- If you have angina, it is moderate and stable.
- If you had a heart attack, between two and six weeks have elapsed since the event.
- If you have class II (moderate) congestive heart failure or a left ventricular ejection fraction lower than 40 percent. (*Ventricular ejection fraction* refers to the ratio of blood your left ventricle pumps to the amount remaining in the ventricle afterward. A normal ejection fraction is roughly between 50 and 60 percent; that is, the ventricle pumps out between 50 and 60 percent of the blood that filled it prior to contraction.)
- If you have peripheral arterial disease (a condition in which the arteries channeling oxygenated blood to the legs, lower abdomen, arms, neck, or head are diseased), a history of stroke, or transient ischemic attacks (which occur when the heart cannot pump enough blood to satisfy the body's oxygen demands; also known as TIAs), or other consequences of atherosclerosis.

If the above-described conditions resemble your own, you are probably at **moderate risk** of suffering cardiac complications due to sex. If you are at moderate risk your cardiac condition is uncertain, and you should pursue further testing, evaluation, or rehabilitation before resuming sexual relations. The test results may lead your physician to assign you to either the high- or low-risk group.

INTERPRETING THE QUESTIONNAIRE: ARE YOU AT HIGH RISK?

You are at **high risk** of cardiac danger from sexual activity if these conditions apply to you:

- You have unstable angina. This means your angina has only recently struck, or is severe, worsening rapidly, or resisting treatment. When this is the case, you are at higher risk for a heart attack during sex or any kind of exertion because your heart's ability to keep up with your body's needs is exceeded by even mild physical activity. Contrary to traditional medical practice, doctors are now telling heart patients *not* to take sublingual nitrates—nitroglycerin tablets under the tongue—if they experience angina-related pain during sex. Rather, if pain occurs, it is wise to stop what you are doing and call your doctor.

It is also important to note that angina can manifest itself as pain in areas other than the chest. Pain may also grab the left shoulder or snake down the inside of the left arm; through the back; in the jaw, throat, or teeth; and sometimes down the right arm. In some cases, people describe the sensation as one of discomfort rather than pain.[34]

Rather than prescribing nitroglycerin to control your angina, your physician will probably advise you to consider other therapies, such as taking a beta-blocking drug and reversing your cardiac risk factors by losing weight, quitting smoking, and so on.[35]

- You have high blood pressure and are not taking medication to control it.
- You have class III to IV—severe to very severe—congestive heart failure.
- If you had a heart attack, it occurred within the last two weeks.
- If you have arrhythmias, particularly ventricular arrhythmias induced by exercise or sex. If you have an ICD or pacemaker, you're in luck—these devices eliminate this risk factor.
- If you have cardiomyopathy, a general term meaning dysfunction of the heart muscle. Scientists haven't done much research into how sexual activity affects people with this condition, but we do know that certain forms of cardiomyopathy are associated with fainting (syncope), and sudden death during or after physical exertion.
- If you have moderate to severe valve disease, particularly aortic stenosis (narrowing of the aortic valve). Although we don't have much information about the risks of sex for these patients, we do know that significant aortic stenosis is associated with sudden death.

If you are a high-risk patient, your condition is serious or unstable enough that sexual activity may be hazardous to your heart. You should speak with your cardiologist before resuming sexual relations or if you are considering treatment for sexual problems. This is of critical importance because certain medications, such as those which aid erection by causing vasodilation (expansion of a blood vessel's diameter to facilitate blood flow), can have profound effects on a less-than-healthy heart. All sexual activity must wait either until your cardiac condition is stabilized or your physician decides it is safe for you to resume sexual activity (or both).

WHEN IT'S SAFE TO RESUME SEX, PLEASE PACE YOURSELF

These risk profiles will clue you in to what your physician is looking for when he or she assesses if sex will be safe for your heart. I emphasize that this is not a decision you should make on your own: **Consult your physician before resuming sex.**

Even when your physician says it's safe, I encourage you to take your time and not overdo it. Well-adjusted patients tell me this is the best advice they have for starting on the journey toward living well with heart disease. Don't worry that your interest in sex is gone forever, never to return. Be realistic—when you suffer a cardiac event or undergo surgery, or both, you're also likely to experience varying degrees of fatigue, fear, anxiety, depression, and physical discomfort, including disheartening, drug-related sexual side effects.

You need to find your comfort level—both yours and your partner's. Most couples find it best to resume sex slowly. Spend time holding, caressing, and perhaps massaging each other (more about this later). Even if your physician has recommended that you avoid sex, don't deny yourself, your intimate partner, and your loved ones physical affection—sitting close, holding hands, touching, hugging, and kissing. Now more than ever, you need the comfort that comes with loving affection and support.

"OH, I'M GETTING OLD!" (AND OTHER FINE WHINES)

While you're wending your way through this sex-after-heart-disease maze, remember that growing older ushers in a variety of medical and sexual side effects of its own. Menopause, arthritis, prostate problems—conditions associated with aging as well as heart illness—can render sex uncomfortable. People tend to make one of two mistakes: either they overestimate the effect of aging on their sex lives, or they underestimate it. Whichever camp you fall into, I advise a balanced approach. First, don't believe the myth that, once those first pinches of salt season the pepper of your hair, you're doomed to rock on the porch of your former passionate self, clinging to fading memories of your hot-blooded youth. Most people say they enjoy sex well into their seventies, some into their eighties, and a few even beyond that.

On the other hand, it's also true that aging alters every aspect of how the body works, and that includes sexual response. As we age, sexual response becomes more elongated. We need more direct sexual stimulation for longer periods of time to achieve climax, and orgasm is likely to be less explosive and more generalized than when we were younger. The sex drive may lessen, and the amount of time between orgasms, also known as the rest or refractory period, usually lengthens.

"SEX WAS DIFFERENT BEFORE
I STARTED TAKING THIS MEDICINE"

Medications can change sexual response, and they affect people in different ways. Physicians cannot accurately predict which drugs will produce sexual side effects in one patient compared to another. Many patients try different medications until they and their doctors agree on a combination that does the most good and least harm. A commonsense approach will help you and your loved ones better understand how your medications might be affecting you.

Breaking the medication side effects code can make anyone's head spin, my own included, but it's worth the investment of at least a few pages. To help you keep track of this discussion, take a look at the Appendix, which provides information about the behavioral, psychological, and sexual side effects of numerous cardiac and psychotropic drugs.

As the Appendix shows, many drugs prescribed to treat heart illness as well as conditions that may occur with it (hypertension and depression, for instance) can compromise your ability to become aroused and achieve orgasm, as well as reduce your sex drive. And it may not surprise you to hear that powerful medications such as those used to control heart rhythms can interfere with sexual response. But we now know that even some medications that do not otherwise have many noticeable side effects—for instance, lipid-lowering drugs, which help reduce blood cholesterol levels—can interfere with sexual arousal. Statins, a category of lipid-regulating medications, are both extremely effective and more than likely to cause erectile difficulties in men who take them (see page 252). But there may be a silver lamé lining to this not-so-sexy cloud: new research strongly suggests that, in addition to reducing cholesterol levels, statins may be effective at treating multiple sclerosis and reducing the risk for both Alzheimer's disease and cancer.[36] Even so, the medicines that affect the sex lives of most heart patients are those that treat hypertension and depression.

ANTIHYPERTENSIVE MEDICATIONS

Many antihypertensive drugs interfere with both male and female sexual response by inhibiting the expansion of blood vessels needed for arousal. Thiazide diuretics and beta-blockers present the most problems.[37] But scientists are developing new formulas that control blood pressure without interfering with sexual response. Alpha-blockers and calcium channel blockers cause fewer sexual problems than traditional antihypertensive drugs. And a new, albeit costly class of remedies for hypertension after heart attack called angiotensin-converting enzyme, or ACE, inhibitors, seems to cause the fewest sexual side effects of all.

Moreover, recent research into the connection between drugs and sexual response suggests that medication may not always be guilty as charged. The Treatment of Mild Hypertension Study (TOMHS) [38] is the most comprehensive investigation to date of long-term effects of blood pressure medications on sexual functioning. The study tracked the effects of anti-hypertensive drugs on the sexual functioning of nine hundred men and women over four years, and found the negative side effects surprisingly low.

While there were indeed cases of impaired sexual response among the participants, the study called attention to an important point: people who have moderate to severe hypertension, cardiovascular illness, or both, who are experiencing sexual problems, and taking antihypertensive drugs, may be suffering more from the effects of the illnesses than the side effects of the medications. For this reason, although changing your medication or dosage may lessen the side effects, experts say it probably won't restore you to full sexual functioning. Instead, it is important that you treat your sexual problems directly, either with counseling, with medication prescribed specifically for that purpose, or both.

ANTIDEPRESSANT MEDICATIONS

As I noted in Chapter 7, selective serotonin reuptake inhibitor antidepressants, or SSRIs, are considered medically safe for heart patients. Unfortunately, they do blunt sexual response in both men and women, muting desire and prompting orgasmic dysfunction, impotence, and ejaculation disturbances. The news isn't all bad, though, as there are some excellent antidepressants that are as effective as SSRIs but less detrimental to sexual response.

Two of these are nefazodone (Serzone) and bupropion (Wellbutrin, Zyban).* In a landmark study, psychiatrist Harry Croft and colleagues compared a sustained-release form of bupropion (Wellbutrin SR) with sertraline, a powerful SSRI marketed as Zoloft.[39] The drugs were equally effective at relieving depression, but Wellbutrin SR caused significantly fewer sexual side effects than Zoloft. In a follow-up study, doctors administered Wellbutrin SR to women who were not depressed but did suffer from

---

* I will introduce a medication first by its generic name and then by its brand name(s), in parentheses.

low sex drive. The results of this study suggested that this medication might be useful in enhancing sexual desire for women.[40]

So, if you're a heart patient who needs an antidepressant and wants a sex life, you'd want to stay away from SSRIs and take either bupropion or nefazodone instead, right? Well, maybe yes, and maybe no. People who take these drugs tend to put on weight, and extra weight overtaxes the heart. Bupropion, which is chemically different from other antidepressants and used as a smoking deterrent as well as a mood enhancer, has been known to cause seizures in people who are prone to them. And in sertraline's favor, a study recently found Zoloft to be safe specifically for heart attack survivors.[41] As I said earlier, sex for heart patients isn't simple; it's got more angles than a geometry class.

Also, we still have a lot to learn about how these antidepressants affect the body. One preliminary study (a study conducted on a small number of subjects to determine the feasibility of doing a more extensive one) evaluated the cardiovascular effects of bupropion in thirty-six patients suffering from depression and either congestive heart failure, ventricular arrythmias, or conduction disturbance (irregularity of the heart's electrical impulses).[42] Happily, the bupropion did not have any marked negative effects, which bodes well for the future of sustained-release Wellbutrin. I hear from my patients that this medication eases depression while inflicting fewer sexual side effects than others they have tried. Still, as with SSRIs, large, long-term, controlled studies of the cardiovascular effects of these other medications have not yet been completed, so we don't know how they are likely to affect most cardiac patients. (Is your head spinning yet? Don't forget the Appendix.)

PRODUCTS THAT ENHANCE SEXUAL RESPONSE

If you stopped ten people on the street between the ages of twenty and ninety, chances are good that none of them could tell you what sildenafil citrate is used for. But if you asked them about Viagra, they'd give you an earful. Viagra is a small blue diamond-shaped tablet that seems to be everywhere—in print ads, TV commercials, even an episode of *Law & Order*. But while Viagra—the brand name under which sildenafil citrate is marketed—may be the most heavily advertised sex-enhancing product, it isn't the only one. In the last few years, various products for enhancing male and female sexual response have come on the market; by the time this volume appears, there will no doubt be more. These new remedies were developed with the rationale that many sexual arousal difficulties stem from impaired blood flow to the penis or vagina and clitoris; each of the remedies works by aiding and abetting that flow.

AROUSAL-ENHANCING HELP FOR WOMEN

While research into women's sexual problems still lags behind that of men's, the pace is picking up. As of this writing, there are no FDA-approved pharmacological treatments for female sexual dysfunction. However, researchers are studying Viagra's potential for helping women and may have found the answer by the time you read these words.[43] And in spring 2002, scientists at the American Urological Association's annual meeting announced two promising treatments for female sexual arousal disorder (FSAD).[44]

The first is an ointment containing a solution of alprostadil, a drug traditionally used to treat male impotence. When the ointment is applied to the clitoris and allowed to spread to surrounding tissue, it stimulates blood flow to the vaginal area and enhances sexual arousal. If you think this treatment might be helpful to you, ask your physician about it—**unless you are a woman of childbearing age, as alprostadil will affect the development of a fetus's heart.**[45] (At this time, there is no evidence that alprostadil adversely affects a woman's heart, whether or not she is pregnant.)

Consequently, men must also be careful if they are taking alprostadil (marketed for erectile dysfunction under the brand names Caverject, Edex, and Muse and administered by injection into the penis or insertion into the urethra), as it passes into semen. If you are a man taking this drug, you must wear a condom if you engage in sexual relations with a pregnant woman.

The second new treatment to be unveiled by the AUA is a lightweight, battery-operated suction device marketed under the name of Eros Therapy that works directly upon the clitoris. When the Eros Therapy is turned on, it creates a gentle vacuum, increasing blood flow to the genital area and improving a woman's ability both to become sexually aroused and to achieve orgasm.

Both the ointment and the vacuum pump have great potential, but remember that they are still in early stages of development and their effects on heart patients are yet to be determined. I advise women taking blood thinners to be especially careful about using any suction device, as it could lead to bruising. Proceed with enthusiasm and caution, and check with your physician.

BEWARE OF EPHEDRINE AND EPHEDRA!

Both female and male heart patients should also be extremely cautious when dealing with ephedrine, a chemical originally extracted from the Chinese ma huang plant and now synthetically produced. Ephedrine is a key component of ephedra—the broader term by which it is commonly identified and the term I shall use here—and is heavily marketed as the active ingredient in dietary weight-loss supplements that have become wildly popular among people attracted to herb-based medicinals. It has also been used since the 1920s in over-the-counter cold and allergy remedies because of its effectiveness as a nasal decongestant. Many people—especially athletes—take ephedra because of its amphetamine-like effects, which can perk you up if you're dragging with a head cold, catapult your energy through the roof if you're not, and also blunt your appetite.

Ephedra has also been touted as something of an aphrodisiac for women,[46] but the honeymoon is over: after years of suspicion, we now have proof that **ephedra is dangerous,** having been implicated in a host of serious medical problems, including heart arrythmia, stroke, psychotic episodes, and even death. The Food and Drug Administration had been unsuccessfully trying for years to restrict ephedra use until February 18, 2003, when Steve Bechler, a twenty-three-year-old pitcher for the Baltimore Orioles, died of heatstroke during a workout in Florida after having used a weight-loss supplement that contained ephedra. Suddenly people were listening and, within weeks, federal officials proposed that warning labels be placed on dietary supplements containing ephedra. As I write this, the FDA is deciding whether to ban it.

How do ephedra's risks compare to those of other herbal products? They are much, much greater: in 2001, 64 percent of all adverse reactions to herbal remedies in the United States were traced to products containing ephedra, even though these products constituted *less than 1 percent of all herbal product sales.*[47] You don't have to be a statistician to see that you have a much higher risk of suffering adverse side effects when you use ephedra than when you use other herbs. The cardiac risks of taking ephedra include coronary artery constriction, vasospasm (sudden decrease in internal diameter of a blood vessel), cardiac arrhythmia, heart attack, and hypertension-related stroke.[48]

Don't be lulled into complacency by labels that proclaim a product is "all natural," "organic," or "botanical"—that doesn't mean it's safe. Ephedrine was originally extracted from a plant, so it's natural, organic, botanical, **and probably hazardous to your heart.** So, whether you're a man or a woman, do not take ephedrine, ephedra, or a non-FDA-approved product related to either of them—*Ephedra sinica, Sida cordifolia,* epitonin, or any of the myriad dietary supplement that contain variations—unless your physician is aware you are taking it and is monitoring your progress.

AROUSAL-ENHANCING HELP FOR MEN

As this paperback edition goes to press, sildenafil citrate, marketed as Viagra, is still the only FDA-approved drug for erectile dysfunction whose cardiovascular effects have been adequately researched. But there may soon be more: two new drugs, vardenafil (to be marketed as Levitra) and tadalafil (to be marketed as as Cialis) are poised for FDA approval in late 2003 and look very promising for heart patients. Advance publicity for Levitra alleges that it works quickly, helping some patients achieve erections in as little as fifteen minutes; Cialis's manufacturer says its effects last longer than those of other medications, in some cases as long as thirty-six hours.[49]

For now, however, Viagra is the main event. It works by increasing the effects of nitric oxide, a chemical released in the penis during sexual stimulation which in turn releases an enzyme that increases blood flow to the penis, producing an erection.

Viagra is the most widely prescribed drug for treating ED. It is also the most discussed and, in some circles of heart patients, the most feared. This is because of a 1999 news story that reported that 377 Viagra users had died of cardiovascular complications ostensibly related to the medication. While the story's implications warrant a variety of responses, I don't believe fear should be one of them, and I'm in good company.

Robert A. Kloner of the Heart Institute at the University of Southern California in Los Angeles has offered a comprehensive and thoughtful analysis of the anxiety surrounding these deaths.[50] Writing in *The American Journal of Cardiology,* Dr. Kloner tells us that, between March 1998 and February 1999, about 9 million prescriptions for Viagra were filled by about 4.5 million men. During this time, 377 deaths due to cardiovascular complications were reported among this group. Of these, 219 were due to MI, arrhythmia, or cardiac arrest, 140 were sudden deaths, and eighteen were due to stroke. Dr. Kloner notes that over half the men died within four to five hours of using Viagra, with about half those deaths occurring during or just after they had engaged in sexual intercourse.

To keep these figures in perspective, you must realize that the average number of deaths among four and a half million male heart patients over an eleven-month period is far, far higher than the number of men who died while using Viagra. Dr. Kloner cites American Heart Association statistics that say about 185 Caucasian and 275 African-American men—a total of 460—per million die from heart disease *each month*. In contrast, the death rate among men who filled Viagra prescriptions was only about 8.5 per million per month—a much lower figure.

With these data in mind, and buttressed by findings of scientists who studied Viagra's effects on men with diabetes or high blood pressure,[51] Dr. Kloner concluded that Viagra is safe for men with chronic but stable heart disease.

But read on! It is also true that **you should not use Viagra in either of two circumstances:**

- **If you are a sedentary male with multiple risk factors**
- **If you are taking nitrates in any form**

If you don't engage in physical exercise and have multiple risk factors—for example, if you smoke, or are obese, or have diabetes—abruptly resuming sexual activity is just as dangerous as heaving yourself off the couch and into a vigorous exercise session. If you're an inactive person and plunge back into sexual activity, you burden your heart with increased oxygen demands. In addition, the excitement of resuming sex may stimulate your sympathetic nervous system and load even more stress on your heart. If you're physically out of shape and haven't had sexual relations in a while, you would be better off easing gradually into sex rather than using Viagra to induce an artificially intense physical reaction your heart may not be ready to handle.

The second warning about Viagra is that it doesn't mix well with nitrates. Experts agree that **combining Viagra with any organic nitrate can lead to large, life-threatening drops in blood pressure.**[52] This class of medications includes nitroglycerin (marketed under a variety of brand names; see the Appendix), isosorbide mononitrate and isosorbide dinitrate (antiangina medications), as well as other nitrate medications.

Also in this group is amyl nitrate, an arousal intensifier long used in the gay community and popularly dispensed in breakaway capsules known as poppers, whose contents are inhaled. Taking Viagra and chasing it with poppers could have disastrous results. The 1999 American College of Cardiology and American Heart Association consensus statement warned people not to ingest any substance containing nitrates within twenty-four hours of taking Viagra.[53]

Finally, even if your physician says Viagra is safe for you, bear in mind that it can cause bothersome if not dangerous side effects such as headache, flushing, breathlessness, and abnormal vision.

Also, Viagra has not been systematically tested in patients with severe, recently diagnosed heart disease. This would include patients with unstable angina or those who have suffered a heart attack in the last six months, and those who have had a stroke or life-threatening arrhythmia. Nor are there complete studies of Viagra's effects on men with congestive heart failure or borderline low blood volume or low blood pressure (hypotension).[54] Finally, substances similar to Viagra have been found to cause muscle damage elsewhere in the body. While we have no evidence that Viagra damages muscle tissue, the drug is still relatively new and its long-term effects on the myocardium—the middle layer of the heart wall—have not yet been evaluated.[55]

Still, evidence continues to mount that Viagra is effective in treating men who have both coronary artery disease and erectile difficulties. So, should you use it? The answer to that question hinges on your answers to these: What are your risk factors for experiencing another cardiac event? Are you obese, do you smoke, are you sedentary? (If so, your risk when engaging in sexual activity may be fairly high.) When you've evaluated your risks, consider whether they are acceptable to you and your partner. Talk with your doctor about Viagra; ask what his or her patients have said about it. Then talk with your partner; discuss the potential risks and benefits.

OTHER OPTIONS FOR MEN AND WOMEN

In addition to these remedies, we now have medical treatments that aid sexual response. These include:

- Medication injected into the penis or applied topically to the penis or vaginal area (a few were mentioned earlier).

- Surgery to bypass clogged arteries leading to the pelvis or repair damaged veins needed to retain blood in the penis.

- A penile implant, a rigid, flexible, or inflatable device surgically placed in the penile shaft to produce an erection.

- A vacuum suction device for men, which draws blood into the penis. The user then places a constrictive ring similar to a large rubber band at the base of the penis to retain the blood and maintain erection.

- A vacuum suction device for women (described earlier).

- For women and men, hormone replacement therapies (HRT) that enhance sexual response. While physicians have been enthusiastically recommending HRT for some patients—especially menopausal women—for many years, they are now reconsidering. In July 2002, a large HRT study was abruptly halted amid findings of increased cardiovascular and breast cancer risks for women taking a combination of estrogen and progestin. It will be some time before we know whether estrogen alone will provide benefits that outweigh the risks of developing other ailments. Be sure to consult your physician and read up on the subject before making a decision about whether hormone replacement therapy is right for you.

MORE TREATMENTS, WITH SOME RESERVATIONS

The good news is that each of these treatments has something to offer. The not-so-good news is that not all of them have been examined for their effects on heart patients, and some of them do pose risks for some people:

- Yohimbine, an alkaloid derived from the bark of the African yohimbé tree, is purported to be an aphrodisiac and has been used to enhance erection. However, I never recommend yohimbine for several reasons: its effectiveness has been questioned by the American Urological Association; its side effects include increased pulse rate and blood pressure, palpitations, and anxiety, and it hasn't been clinically evaluated for use by heart patients.[56]

- Penile injections of papaverine, phentolamine, or prostaglandin E1 have helped men achieve erection but may cause blood pressure to drop and interfere with liver function, which is vital to the body's ability to manage cholesterol. A physician may also rule out penile injections for a man who is taking anticlotting medication.

- Vacuum suction devices are generally safe, but the constricting rubber ring placed on the penis after using one may cause problems if the man has severe blood vessel disease. Such patients should leave the ring in place no longer than fifteen minutes. Also, if you are taking anticlotting medication, you may bruise excessively when using a vacuum suction device.

Should you try one or more of these treatments? Quite possibly, but you should base your decision on a thoughtful evaluation of your medical and psychological condition. Everyone is different; what works for one person may not work for you.

WHAT YOU CAN DO TO RECLAIM YOUR SEX LIFE

Once you know what your risks are and your physician says that sex is safe for your heart, you can stop thinking so much and start having fun. The point is to take responsibility for reviving your sex life: it may not come back on its own, much as you would like it to, and you may have to put effort into getting it back. Intimacy and erotic pleasure are fundamental to life; to live without them is to forsake an essential aspect of your nature. Here are some things for patients to bear in mind:

- **Anxiety about the ability to respond sexually is normal and affects nearly all heart patients.** It usually passes with time.

- **Things might not go perfectly the first time (or even after).** You must learn to develop confidence in your ability to enjoy sex even though you have heart illness. Confidence might not come on its own; you must practice. But when it comes to sex, practice seldom makes perfect. All of us—whether we have heart disease or not—sometimes have problems with sex. Accept that sex is a part of life, not the whole shebang but a part of it, and try not to overreact.

- **Some signs of sexual arousal—rapid heartbeat, shallow breathing— can mimic symptoms of cardiovascular problems.** Don't think you're having a heart attack if you're just turned on.

- **Pace yourself.** If the idea of self-stimulation is acceptable to you, you might try a solo erotic experience to restore confidence that you can indeed become sexually aroused and live to enjoy it.

- **You're not the only one with sexual issues.** Your partner is probably anxious too, perhaps more than you are. Talk about your concerns and anxieties, and accept that learning to have sex now that one of you has heart disease is new territory for both of you.

- **Think of sex as a particularly enjoyable workout, and remember these commonsense guidelines:**

  - **Don't make love in excessive heat or cold or after a long evening of heavy eating or drinking,** as you will place undue strain on your heart.

  - **After a meal, wait at least ninety minutes before having sex.** When you eat, your brain tells your heart to pump blood to the digestive system. If you make love soon after a meal, your heart will have to work harder to get the blood everywhere it needs to go—an unnecessary strain.

  - **While spontaneity is a powerful aphrodisiac, there's something to be said for planning.** If you're thinking about making love, wait to initiate sex until you and your partner are both relaxed, and choose positions that do not strain your surgical wounds.

- **If you are not in a monogamous relationship, choose your partners wisely.** The more comfortable you are with a lover, the more likely it is that your body will aid and abet your sexual intentions.

- **Rest for a while before you make love,** and afterward as well.

- **Don't abruptly plunge into moderate to vigorous exercise of any sort if you have been sedentary for a long time—and this includes sex!** Start slowly, increase your exertion level gradually, and get into shape. Even if you're not a heart patient, you'll do well to remember this.

- **Do not attempt sexual relations when you are emotionally raw or overwrought.**

- **Use positions that are comfortable for both you and your partner.**[57]

- **If you've had surgery,** you may find sex easier if your partner is on top during the early stages of wound healing. This helps keep pressure off your chest and leg wounds.

- **If either you or your partner is significantly overweight, consider a rear-entry, standing position.** This removes the need to have a heavy partner on top. And, of course, if you favor the missionary position, it helps if the overweight partner is on the bottom.

- **To prevent shortness of breath, try lying side by side facing each other during sex.** Or try the spooning position, where you also lie side by side but face the same direction. This encourages more leisurely lovemaking.

- **Select from a varied menu of sexual experiences; don't always go for the early-bird special.** Not every encounter need involve athletic intercourse and explosive orgasms. Be generous in the pleasures you offer each other and gracious when responding to your partner's erotic offerings, even if what you receive is not exactly what you'd hoped for.

- **Never mix nitrates with sildenafil citrate (Viagra) or any arousal-enhancing medication or formula.**

- **Never take ephedrine or any of its non-FDA-approved derivatives—*Ephedra sinica, Sida cordifolia,* or epitonin—unless you have discussed it with your doctor and are under medical supervision.**

- **If you have a history of heart rhythm disturbances or are concerned about developing one, avoid anal intercourse.**

- **Do *not* stop taking *any* cardiac medication because of sexual side effects.** Instead, talk to your doctor. He or she may be able to prescribe a different medication with less debilitating side effects.

Here are some tips I offer to both my patients and their partners:

- **There's more to intimacy than sex.** Your mutual anxiety about sex and heart illness will lessen as you both become comfortable discussing sex, being affectionate, and relaxing together as you focus on intimacies beyond intercourse and orgasm. Be open. Be playful. Be loving. Relax, and delight in each other.

- **Take time to get to know each other again.** Start by trading back rubs (or foot rubs or whatever kinds of rubs you favor). If you are self-conscious about your surgery scars, try holding each other while still wearing your nightclothes. When you're ready, ask your partner to apply lotion to your scars; this will desensitize your anxiety. Then, little by little, allow these affectionate sessions to grow sexually playful. Yes, there is a point where you must leap into nothingness and trust the person you love to catch and hold and cherish you, scars and all. The sooner you take the leap toward physical affection, the sooner you will heal. Rather than focus on intercourse and orgasm—the goal-oriented approach to sex—luxuriate instead in the process of lovemaking. Surrender to the journey by using all your senses: sight, smell, taste, hearing, and touch. Savor the delicious sensations you may usually be too preoccupied to notice. This will help you relax, inspire affection for your partner, and in turn persuade your body to cooperate by becoming sexually aroused. Try this:
  Look at your bodies as you are touching and making love, or close your eyes and picture yourselves in your mind. Taste your partner's skin. Notice the texture of your partner's hair. Feel the warmth of your bodies coming together. Listen to the sounds you make. When your consciousness is saturated with these sensations, there is no room for worry of the sort that could compromise your body's sexual response.

IF YOU HAVE CHEST PAIN DURING SEX

When you're in the throes of passion is not the ideal time to pull away and discuss strategies for dealing with a cardiac emergency. It's better to take ten minutes now to decide what you will do should you have chest pain, or pain elsewhere, during sex. If this happens, use your common sense:

- Tell your partner you're in pain.
- Stop what you're doing and sit or lie comfortably.
- Cardiologists now recommend that you not use nitroglycerin to relieve chest pain during sex. Instead, they say you should stop what you were doing when the pain began and call your physician.

- If the pain continues for more than fifteen or twenty minutes, call 911 or get to either an emergency room or urgent care facility.

Even if you get through an episode of sex-related chest pain without having to see a doctor, **discuss the event with your doctor as soon as possible.** In fact, I recommend that you call your doctor if you experience any of these symptoms:

- Rapid pulse, rapid breathing, or shortness of breath for twenty minutes or longer after sex
- Angina during sex
- Irregular heartbeat or palpitations (fluttering) for twenty minutes or longer after sex
- Trouble sleeping after sex or feeling very tired the day after

HOW TO DISCUSS SEX WITH YOUR DOCTOR

Sex is a funny thing: it's all around us—in the movies and the news, on TV, in ads and commercials—and we think about it a lot more than we're willing to admit. But when it comes to talking about it, well, that's another story. Yet you *must* learn to talk about it if you've got heart disease and want to reclaim your sex life. You have to be able to look your doctor in the eye and describe your symptoms, feelings, and fears, and articulate the questions you'd been too shy to ask.

You can help yourself initiate such a discussion by preparing for it well in advance of your appointment. If you don't, you're likely to become self-conscious, cloak your embarrassment in a vague description of the problem, nod and accept what the doctor says, even if he or she hasn't adequately answered your questions, and leave the office just as anxious and uncertain as you were when you walked in. Even worse, you may misinterpret what the doctor says—or doesn't say—and work yourself up into a state of high and utterly unwarranted anxiety.

Start preparing for such a discussion by making an appointment to talk with your physician apart from your examination. Let the scheduling clerk know there are some issues you would like to discuss with the doctor, and ask for an appointment to do so. Otherwise, she or he may assume that yours is a routine "get-'em-in, get-'em-out fast" sort of visit, and you will be rushed. Your physician would be the first one to tell you that managed care guidelines require doctors to see many more patients each day than they can comfortably serve and that they must rush through appointments. While you probably can't reform the system, you can state up front that you need some time with the doctor, a physician's assistant, or a nurse.

Next, take a piece of paper and a few moments to jot down a detailed analysis of your problem or concern. Be honest; have the courage to put your worry into words. Then think about ways to articulate your thoughts and feelings.

Here are some questions your doctor is likely to ask and some ways you might phrase your responses:

DOCTOR: What kind of sexual changes have you noticed?
PATIENT: I have less desire than I used to.
PATIENT: I have trouble getting turned on sexually.
PATIENT: I can get aroused, but I have trouble reaching orgasm.
PATIENT: I have trouble maintaining a full erection.

DOCTOR: When did you first notice these changes?
PATIENT: I was doing fine before I started taking this medicine.
PATIENT: I was doing fine until the heart attack (or the surgery, or until I found out I had heart disease).
PATIENT: Actually, things were happening for a while before the heart attack (or the surgery, or before I started taking the medication).

DOCTOR: Are you comfortable with your body?
PATIENT: I'm not sure I know what you mean.
DOCTOR: What I mean is, how do you feel about your body now? Are you able to allow your partner to see you undressed?
PATIENT: Yes, I guess I'm comfortable with my body. I wish I didn't have this scar running down my chest, but it could have been a lot worse.
PATIENT: No, I feel self-conscious about my scars.
PATIENT: No. I don't trust my body since the heart attack.
PATIENT: No. I'm more conscious than ever of being overweight. I don't like taking off my clothes in front of anyone.

DOCTOR: Is intercourse pleasurable for you, or do you have discomfort?
PATIENT: It's not as easy as it used to be; I seem to be too dry.
PATIENT: No, it's not quite right. I can get an erection, but it's painful.

PATIENT: Everything is working the way it's supposed to, but my incisions hurt.

Here are some more questions your doctor may ask; you can fill in your own responses:

- Have you ever had chest pain during sex or afterward? If so, in what circumstances?
- Are there circumstances in which sex goes more smoothly for you than in others?
- Are you nervous about having sex?
- Are you depressed?
- How do you feel after having sex, physically and emotionally?
- Can you and your wife (husband, partner) talk easily about your relationship?
- Do you feel your partner is afraid to have sex?
- Has your sex life been affected by menopause, either yours or your partner's? If so, how?
- Have you had prostate problems?

Your mission in this meeting is to steer the discussion in the direction you want it to go. Come to the appointment with a list of the issues you want to bring up; don't entrust them to memory. The talk may meander from the original topic, which is fine, but you may get sidetracked and run out of time before you've covered the material you came to discuss.

Remember: this is a critical component of your health care. Your intimate life is not a luxury you can afford to forego, and you owe it to yourself to consult with a physician who embraces this philosophy. Do not allow a doctor to patronize you, nor should you tolerate condescending comments such as "You can't expect sex to last forever. You're lucky to be alive at your age, after a heart attack like that." Sex *can* last a very long time; in some cases, all of your life. If your physician tries to persuade you otherwise, consider finding a different doctor.

Sexual performance problems are not minor side effects of medication, aging, or your condition that you should dismiss with nary a care. If your physician implies this, you might say, "Doctor, the only minor side effects are those that happen to other people. It's my life we're talking about, and this is very important to me."

If it's important to you, make sure your physician knows about it, and treats you accordingly.

Chapter Ten

BELIEVE IN SOMETHING
GREATER THAN YOURSELF

Every thriving heart patient I have known over the past twenty-five years has something in common with the others: all have said that, in one way or another, the illness forced them to look beyond themselves and seek a higher purpose in life.

Most have said their awakening began with a sense of regret over how much time they'd wasted ignoring what meant most to them: after years of struggling with their daily routines, heart illness heightened their awareness of a more profound reality. For some, this meant noticing the beauty of their loved ones; for others, having a greater appreciation of everyday pleasures and moments of peace.

So many people have told me the same story: after years of skimming across life's surface, heart illness brought them to their knees. Men and women who were too busy, too pragmatic, too rational to connect with their spiritual cores find themselves gazing inward, outward, and upward when their lives are on the line.

It's natural to look beyond your own life when you fear it may be torn from you. Doing so broadens your perspective. You begin to see yourself and others in a clear, new light that illuminates some blessings you may have taken for granted, some ways to correct the course of your life, and some questions you must consider, even if there are no answers:

- "When I learned I needed a bypass, I started praying to a God I hadn't turned to since I was thirteen. Aren't I a hypocrite?" (There is an answer to this one, and it's No!)

- "I've had this strange feeling that, in a way, the heart attack was a relief; that now I'm allowed to take care of myself, sometimes before I tend to others. Am I being selfish?"

- "I've been having morbid thoughts lately. I keep picturing myself dying, and then no one shows up at the funeral. Why am I doing this?"

- "Since the heart attack, I've had this weird compulsion to call up all the people I've ever been a jerk to and tell them I'm sorry. What's this all about?"

It's about reconciliation with others and oneself, coming to terms with life, and looking for a higher purpose in your existence.

I am writing this chapter not to persuade you to get religion but to encourage you to direct your gaze upward and outward, beyond your medical history, your symptoms, and the limits of what you know, toward the realm of what is greater than yourself. What gives meaning to *your* life? Maybe it's your partner, and the illness is motivating you to give him or her more of your energy and love. Perhaps it's your work, and you are finding solace and renewal in it. There's something about believing in something that helps people heal, and every heart patient should know it.

THE LANGUAGE OF THE HEART

Straight from the heart . . . my heartfelt thanks . . . what's really in my heart . . . thinking with my heart . . . a soft place in my heart . . . heart and soul . . . follow your heart . . . from the bottom of my heart. These and other sayings remind us that the heart is the seat of the soul: it symbolizes the purity of the self; it is the crucible that shelters the flame of our fiercest and most tender essence.

It's no wonder that heart disease and the image it conjures of a pallid, weakened spirit stirs our vulnerabilities and moves us to examine our lives. Some patients are motivated to heal the wounding their bodies have suffered after years of ill-use. Others respond by imbuing their lives with a higher purpose. Some are unaware of their lives' significance until others awaken them to it.

Examining the principles that govern your life and grant it meaning can lift your spirits but may also be distressing. You may dredge up ancient regrets about lost opportunities and friendships you allowed to wither. You will face your most glaring imperfections. And you may find yourself angry with God or the universe in general because you're suffering.

"I don't understand why this happened to me" is a common refrain of patients who have yet to make peace with themselves. As one man put it, "I've been a good person all my life; I've sacrificed to do what's right by my wife and kids. I always believed that God was just and righteous. But now I'm wondering, why me? What did I do to deserve this? It isn't fair, and I'm angry."

THRIVING WITH HEART DISEASE

This man's faith began to waver just when he needed it most, and I've seen it happen many times. But I've also seen the crisis of serious illness open a person's eyes to the openheartedness of others and awaken a belief in a nurturing higher power.

STANLEY

Stanley, a sixty-three-year-old sales manager for a meatpacking company, was such a person. When he entered the cardiac rehab program, his psychological screening indicated that he was struggling with hostility, and his recent heart attack had transformed this personality trait into a risk factor. His handshake was firm and I was struck by his intense good looks; his nose was finely chiseled, as were the rest of his features, and his dark eyes were unflinching.

As I talked about the dangers of mismanaged anger and hostility, Stanley seemed distracted. He studied a stain on the floor, gazed out the window, squirmed in his chair, then crossed his arms and looked at me accusingly over his eyeglasses. I asked him if he was feeling angry, and the answer didn't surprise me.

"Angry? I've been angry for as long as I can remember. I'm great at figuring out what's wrong with people and letting them know about it. That's what we did in our family; that's probably why we rarely speak to one another, my brothers and me, and why I moved so far away from them.

"But my problems came with me. I've argued with my neighbors, with people at work, with my doctors, even with people at church. It's only since the operation that I've begun to see that I'm the problem.

"You know what did it? The day of the surgery, thirty-two men from my church came and sat with my wife in the waiting room. Thirty-two—they had to bring in extra chairs. When my wife told me that, I . . . I cried. For days, all I could think about was I'd be hard-pressed to name thirty-two people I've been kind to in my entire life. Yet these people came to support me and my family—thirty-two men."

VERA

Vera is a shy, somewhat awkward forty-nine-year-old African American, young to have suffered a heart attack. She is single and the rest of her family lives in another state. A rehab nurse referred her to me when she noticed that Vera seldom interacted with the other patients, remaining instead on the periphery of the banter that seemed to comfort many of the others.

She leaned forward in her chair throughout the session, as if she were struggling to find answers to my questions. When I asked whether she had people to turn to for support as she recovered from her heart attack, she relaxed a bit:

"I work in the cafeteria at the medical school, and my boss has been very understanding about my needing time off to come to rehab. I guess you never know who you can count on to help you.

"Several years ago I joined a church near my house. I've never been much of a churchgoer, but I thought it would be a good idea. I made one new friend there, and a woman I work with is also a member. After my surgery, I was out of circulation for a few weeks. I guess my friend told the minister about my heart attack, and he called a few times to check on me. I appreciated that.

"But I'll never forget that first Sunday when I went back to church. I didn't think anyone there even knew who I was. But five different people came up to say they were glad to see me. Then, right as he was about to start the sermon, the preacher welcomed me back and said they had all been praying for me. Everybody in that church stood up and applauded; they gave me a standing ovation. I'll never forget that for the rest of my life."

SPIRITUALITY, RELIGION, PRAYER, AND HEALTH

Stanley's and Vera's experiences are personal evidence that belonging to a faith community can provide social as well as spiritual support, which is good for cardiovascular health. And there's scientific evidence as well: research shows that people who regularly attend religious services tend to live longer than those who don't. One study of the general population found that people who did not attend services had nearly a 90 percent higher risk of dying during a nine-year period than those who attended services one or more times a week.[1] In fact, those who never attend services live an average of seventy-five years, while those who attend services at least once a week live to an average age of eighty-three.[2]

The data are convincing: eight out of ten studies show that patients with a decided religious commitment are more likely to survive cancer and heart disease and enjoy a higher quality of life and lower levels of anxiety, depression, anger, and substance abuse.[3] We cannot definitively say why this is so,

THRIVING WITH HEART DISEASE

but we do know that praying, meditating, and other forms of mindfulness associated with religious practice soothe the spirit, the body, and the mind, and this makes people healthier.

It also makes them resilient: when illness strikes, many people say they derive strength from their beliefs. Forty percent of Americans over the age of sixty say they turn to religion as a basic energy source when they are hospitalized with a medical illness;[4] 80 percent believe in the power of God or prayer to improve the course of their illness;[5] and, according to one study, 97 percent of surgery patients say that prayer aided their recovery.[6]

ON THE OTHER HAND . . .

This topic is not without controversy. Skeptics say studies that associate religion and healing are imprecise, and that research with high blood pressure patients and heart patients indicates they derived no health benefits from religious involvement.[7]

It is also clear that belief systems that foster guilt and shame in their adherents can damage both mental and physical health, as does the school of thought that interprets illness as retribution, divine or otherwise, for a person's character flaws. Dutiful worshipers of a harsh, unforgiving God suffer more anxiety and depression than those whose deity is more benevolent.[8] People who expect God to solve their problems have higher stress, depression, and suicide rates than those whose beliefs spur them to take responsibility for their lives, albeit with an underlying sense of God's support. And people whose religious fervor becomes compulsive tend to suffer excessive anxiety and dependency and develop more health problems than those who manage not to cross the line between adoration and addiction.[9]

MAINTAIN YOUR PERSPECTIVE

While I don't believe there is an unwavering, concrete correlation between religious commitment and better health, I do believe there are certain things that science can't explain. And I also acknowledge the obvious (and suggest you to do, too): illness is frightening, and when people are frightened they reach for what steadies and heartens them. For many, this means approaching, defining, and embracing their spiritual selves. For most, it involves taking comfort in and drawing strength from a belief system that helps them make sense of life and imbue it with meaning. These beliefs need not be religious in nature; they may be a commitment to an intellectual and emotional ethos as noble and profound as that put forth by any of the great religions. What belief systems have in common is a mechanism by which a human being can grasp, on some level, the meaning of what he or she is going through.

In all my years of counseling heart patients, I've found that the ones who thrive find a way to make sense of their suffering. Some do it by taking shelter in their religious traditions. Others seize the opportunity to mend damaged friendships or take more loving care of themselves. Still others give themselves permission to be still long enough to let life get through to them.

Every thriving patient seems to mature and to grow wiser in the wake of his or her diagnosis. Although they tread different paths to get there, each thriving patient manifests a heightened spiritual sense, or mindfulness, of the infinite world around them and their mysterious place in it.

That's how it was for Sylvia Meyers, a sixty-nine-year-old high school chemistry teacher who had been divorced for many years:

"My rehabilitation has been about healing my life, not just my heart. Over the years, I became so accustomed to being busy that staying busy became my life. At first it was necessary; I was still in my thirties when my husband left and I had two young sons to raise. Each morning as I opened my eyes I'd think, 'What do I need to do today? Do we have milk? What do the boys need for school?'

"Then, when they left home and things quieted down, I thought I'd quiet down, too, but I didn't . . . I couldn't. I'd still be thinking, 'Did I finish my lesson plans? Do I have enough coffee for the morning?' I never paused long enough to just be still and look beyond my circle of obligations.

"The best thing about this diagnosis is that it forced me to take stock of my existence. I think more about what I have, not just what I'm trying to get, and about what I've accomplished, not just what I still need to do. Yesterday, I heard from an old student who went on to get a Ph.D. in chemistry. She wrote to tell me that I was the first woman scientist she'd ever known, and that I actually inspired her to go out and become one herself. I just sat there and pressed that letter to my heart and allowed myself to feel . . . well, I suppose I felt proud. I sat there weeping, but it felt so good, and so real."

It is this heightened sense of the real that betokens contact with your innermost, authentic spirit. To recover fully, open your heart to this part of yourself.

FAITH, RELIGION, AND SPIRIT: WHICH IS WHICH?

Between 10 and 20 percent of Americans say they are spiritual but not religious,[10] while slightly over 50 percent say they are both.[11]

What's the difference? And why even go into it? Because I want you to know that whatever method you use to make sense of your illness, achieve serenity, and stoke the fires of hope, you are not alone.

Some people have an abiding faith in God but seldom attend services or follow the precepts set forth by the religion whose deity they embrace. These people might say that, although they believe in God, they are more spiritual than religious. Religious people, on the other hand, combine a belief in God with participation in rituals and activities sanctioned by a particular faith.

Many people, especially baby boomers in their forties and fifties, describe themselves as spiritual seekers rather than people who believe in God. Although they may feel affection for and connection with the religion in which they were raised, they seldom attend services and prefer to search for meaning by following an individual path rather than the more traveled traditional one. People who think of themselves as spiritual rather than religious might say their souls derive comfort from cultivating inner peace, the profound tranquillity that comes from approaching others with compassion and recognizing and respecting the innate dignity of all living things.

WHAT ARE YOU WAITING FOR?

If you were told today that you only had one year (or six months or two weeks) to live, how would you spend your remaining time? For heart patients and their loved ones, this is more than a brainteasing question; it's a real one. In the best-case scenario, it inspires everyone—patient and family members alike—to reconsider what's really important and reorder their priorities so they may live in greater harmony with their truest selves.

How might you allow this illness help you thrive rather than merely survive? Here are some spiritual prescriptions from various experts combined with a liberal dose of my own:

1. **Take a spiritual inventory.** Both religious and spiritual beliefs can allay your fear of death in numerous ways, not least by fostering a belief in an afterlife or altered state of being in which your soul continues to exist after your body has perished. What is your perception of the transcen-

dent or the divine in everyday life? What beliefs and behaviors spark this connection for you?

I have culled the questions that follow from several psychological inventories designed to help people think more clearly about their spiritual and religious inclinations.[12] They are not meant to reproach you for what you haven't been thinking or feeling, but to stimulate thoughtful inquiry about what soothes your soul and transports you to an exalted state of consciousness:

• Do your beliefs lend a spiritual significance to your illness?

• What fears or concerns are you facing now?

• Is believing in God or a higher power important to you? If you answered yes, how so?

• What is your source of strength and hope during difficult times?

• Does your faith give you strength?

• Do you perform a ritual of any kind that inspires you with joy and elevates you above your daily concerns?

• Does your faith comfort you?

• Does your compassion for others ever override concern for yourself?

• Do you forgive others when they do things you think are wrong?

• Which activities make you feel connected with the universe beyond yourself?

• What experiences grant you serenity and a feeling of inner harmony?

• What helps you feel God's presence in the midst of everyday life?

• Are you grateful for the good in your life?

• Does the beauty of nature touch your spirit?

• Has your illness affected your faith or spiritual beliefs? If so, how?

These questions suggest only a few ways that people transcend the tangible and approach the divine. You may accomplish it by singing, listening to opera, rocking your grandchild, walking in the woods, lavishing affection on your pet, reading, keeping a journal, or in a thousand other ways—including going to church, synagogue, mosque, or wherever you find God.

2. **Be grateful for what you have.** Thriving with heart disease means learning to appreciate all things, great and small, that make your life what it is. To remind yourself that you *are* thriving, take these tips:

• Once a week, write down five things you're thankful for. Start each day by reviewing what you're looking forward to, and end each day by taking stock of what was good and pleasant about it.

- Develop the habit of looking for the good in people.
- Give thanks for simple pleasures such as nourishing food or a dry armchair on a rainy day.
- Remind yourself that each breath is a gift.
- Develop an awareness of the beauty of nature, and appreciate it.
- Contemplate your history and the meaning of your life, knowing that the way you treat others will be your legacy.

3. **Learn to relax.** You can't enjoy your life if you are too stressed to experience it.

- Slow down and practice mindfulness (paying attention). Look within; pray, or meditate, or engage in a meditative activity (for suggestions, see Chapter 6).
- Do one thing at a time.
- Practice breathing deeply—pulling air into your lungs while expanding your belly—to increase your awareness of the moment.

4. **Respond appropriately to disappointment; don't overreact when things don't go the way you want them to.** Wise men and women learn to flow through hard times rather than bog themselves down with regrets. One way to do this is to develop a philosophy that helps you deal with disappointment. Understand that everyone is disappointed at times; disappointment is not an indication of personal or family failure; setbacks are a normal part of living, and illness is an inevitable part of living a long time. And there's always the serenity prayer: *God, grant me serenity to accept the things I cannot change, courage to change the things I can, and wisdom to know the difference.*

5. **Deepen your human connections.** By now you know that I'm convinced that thriving heart patients and healthy, loving relationships go hand-in-hand. Here are a few more reminders:

- **Help others.** People who volunteer in their communities live longer than those who don't.[13]
- **Thank people** for their friendship and caring.
- **Stay in touch** with people who matter to you.
- **Make conversation** with people you encounter in daily life. Ask a colleague how his kids are doing; chat with the pharmacist about your new medication; tell your letter carrier you're glad she's back on the job.
- **Show an interest** in what interests the person you're with, even if you have to pretend a little.

6. **Align your behaviors with your values and goals.** Living out of harmony with your values is toxic. Coping with crisis gives you an opportunity to realign your choices with your values. Here are some ways to do it:

- Ask yourself: "What does happiness mean to *me?*"
- Ask yourself: "What do I need to bring happiness into my life?"
- Make a list of the desires and goals you had when you were a child, an adolescent, a young adult, middle-aged, and now. *Do not judge yourself.* If you dreamed of being a prima ballerina when you were seven but haven't gotten off your tutu since then, so be it: if it was important to you then, write it down now. Then ask yourself:
  - Do these desires and goals still move me?
  - What qualities did I have to develop to pursue and fulfill them?
  - Which of these desires and goals are manifest in my life, and in what ways?
  - Which of them have I yet to achieve?
- Compose a list of the moral and ethical values that govern your life.
  - Are your goals in harmony with these values?
  - Are you devoting sufficient time and energy to the pursuit of your goals?
  - Is your behavior congruent with your goals?
- Ask yourself: "What do I hope to accomplish during my life? Why?"
- Consider: Do you believe your life has a purpose? Why do you think you are here?
- Each week, identify and perform at least one action that brings you closer to fulfilling your life's purpose.
- Happiness is a choice you make, not a commodity bestowed upon you from on high. Learn to focus on the good in your life, and find meaning and wisdom in the mundane parts of living.

7. **Do more of what you truly love to do and less of what you're not crazy about, and eliminate whatever makes you feel angry, sad, or bad (and that includes people).** Surrounding yourself with people who feed your spirit and nourish your soul (and participating in activities that do the same thing) may be the single most powerful way to build resilience and ensure your survival. Here are some ideas:

- Make a list of your favorite simple pleasures.
- Each day, set aside time to enjoy at least one of them. Plan it. Anticipate it. Savor it.

- Make a list of events, activities, and people you dread. Wherever you can, eliminate them from your life.

- Now make a list of people, places, activities, and events that exalt your spirit. Don't let a day go by without seeing or communicating with at least one of these people, visiting one of these places, completing one of these activities, or participating in one of these events.

8. **Forgive others, and seek forgiveness from others.** Few things sever a transcendent connection faster than guilt, shame, and blame, all of which abound in the human breast. None of us escapes unscathed from our humanity; all of us squirm when we relive, in the privacy of our minds, the hateful things we've said and the unkind things we've done— not to mention the lousy things people have done to us.

    As you know by now, this isn't good for your health. Part of thriving with heart disease involves learning to forgive others, to forgive yourself, and to seek forgiveness from others. Both granting and receiving forgiveness helps you let go of past hurts so they can heal and liberate you to take pleasure in your present and your future.

9. **Prepare for the inevitable.** We're here for all too brief a time; all of us will die, no matter how beloved or necessary we are. Family members are particularly adept at tiptoeing on eggshells when it comes to death and dying; everyone knows it's going to happen, but putting it into words seems traitorous, as if talking about it will hasten its arrival or unmask a lack of feeling for the person who is ill. Yet I assure you, heart patients think about death and dying, and yearn to reach closure with the people they love.

    Profound intimacy and meaning will gently fill a relationship when you can discuss your fear of the unknown, of dying, and your hopes for what may await you after this life. Quell the anxieties that can taint your remaining years by getting your affairs in order: your will and financial records, what you'd prefer for a funeral and memorial service, and the many details that could clutter your remaining days with the people you love. Make your wishes known about how you want to be treated near the end of life; write a Durable Power of Attorney for Health Care (also known as a living will) that documents your wishes and names someone to make decisions when you no longer can. If you don't wish to be kept alive by extraordinary means, say so.

10. **Celebrate!** Rejoice in what is good and right in your life. Celebrate and cherish your family. Exult in the gift of yet another morning and the abundant sensations that punctuate the passage of time. While we are still in the quick of life, it is our sacred duty to live it.

PART TWO

❖

THE DOCTOR IS IN:
SPECIAL SESSIONS

Chapter Eleven

LIVING WELL WITH
HEART FAILURE (HF)

More than most diseases, heart failure demands
patient participation.

—MARC SILVER, M.D.[1]

Heart failure. The name itself is ominous, conjuring images of death and dying. Receiving a diagnosis of heart failure leaves many patients thrashing about in anger and despair. And unlike a heart attack or bypass surgery, which typically entails a few periodic follow-up visits with a cardiologist and an occasional hospital stay, a diagnosis of heart failure usually means regular visits to the doctor and the hospital.

It used to be that a diagnosis of heart failure meant you didn't have much longer to live. The great news is that this is no longer true. Even though long-standing heart failure does cause irreversible damage, the disease *is* treatable. Most often, doctors treat the condition by relieving the severity of its symptoms, which improves the patient's quality of life. Medical researchers are even suggesting that some damaged heart tissue can be recovered by increasing blood flow to the area.[2]

That's not all. In fall 2002, *The New England Journal of Medicine* published a study that generated a wave of excitement in the medical field. Researchers at the University of Cincinnati discovered that congestive heart failure is linked to two variant genes, giving people with these genes ten times the risk of developing the condition. The discovery may enable doctors to distinguish medications to help these patients and to find people at high risk early enough to halt the progress of the disease. While people without the altered genes can still develop heart failure, the findings have profound implications for both those whose heart failure is genetically linked and for their relatives, who have a higher likelihood of developing the disease.[3] And there's more: at a November 2002 meeting of the American Heart Association, scientists reported that regular phone calls from nurses to heart failure patients at home resulted in 28 percent fewer hospital readmissions and dramatically reduced health care costs. The authors of the study, which was conducted in Argentina, concluded that similar programs—in which medical professionals regularly phone heart failure patients after they leave the hospital to monitor their progress and offer advice—might be implemented in other countries and ease the suffering of millions of people around the world at a minimal cost.[4]

While breakthroughs such as these promise better lives for heart failure patients, the most critical component of living with the condition is **you: your commitment to participate actively in the management of your illness, and to motivate your family members to join the cause.** This means taking your medications as prescribed, monitoring your salt intake, protecting yourself from flu and other upper respiratory illnesses (in other words, by getting a flu shot), and managing your emotions.

You *cannot* live passively with heart failure and hope to do well. It's an unforgiving disease, and will swiftly worsen unless you adopt an assertively optimistic attitude and surround yourself with options that promote your health. Five million Americans have been diagnosed with heart failure— more patients end up in the hospital because of it than because of all cancers *combined*—and if you're one of them, this chapter will suggest ways to live well with the condition.[5] If you don't have heart failure, the information it contains may someday prove useful should you develop the disease.

Which brings us to the next question: *Will* you develop heart failure? You are at risk if you:

- Have had a heart attack
- Have had a heart infection
- Have a heart murmur
- Are overweight
- Have high blood pressure
- Drink heavily, smoke cigarettes, or abuse drugs
- Have diabetes
- Have a family history of heart failure

Having these risk factors doesn't mean you *will* develop heart failure; it means you're *more likely to* develop the condition than someone who doesn't have them.

HEART FAILURE: WHAT IT IS AND WHAT IT ISN'T

Heart failure is a treatable condition. In some cases, it's even reversible. You can start fortifying yourself against the disease by putting it into perspective.

First, know that you are not alone. Nearly 5 million Americans are currently living with heart failure. It is the fastest-growing form of heart disease, with more than 550,000 new cases diagnosed each year. Heart failure strikes equal numbers of men and women (although new cases of heart failure among women have dropped by a third over the last fifty years[6]), and the likelihood of having it increases with age:

- Two percent of Americans between the ages of forty and fifty-nine have it.
- Five percent between sixty and sixty-nine have it.
- Ten percent of Americans seventy and older have it.

The incidence of heart failure among African Americans is 25 percent higher than the figures quoted above.[7]

WHAT DOES HEART FAILURE MEAN?

It means that the heart is not pumping as well as it should because of damage to heart muscle. The term is not meant to imply that the heart fails to beat, but rather that it fails in its primary task, which is to deliver enough oxygen- and nutrient-rich blood to the body. When the heart cannot do this, the body cannot function properly and you're left feeling weak, fatigued, short of breath, or all three.

Heart failure is more a syndrome than a disease. It's a collection of cardiac-related difficulties that arise from a variety of conditions that weaken the heart muscle over time. These may include clogged arteries, high blood pressure, defective heart valves, lung disease, or poorly controlled risk factors such as diabetes and obesity. A heart attack, chronic arrhythmia, or other condition may also damage the heart muscle and set the stage for the development of heart failure. Heart failure may also result from thyroid problems, vitamin B1 deficiency, or anemia, in which case there is usually no underlying cardiomyopathy (damaged heart muscle). There's also some mystery surrounding heart failure; about two out of five cases are diagnosed as being of unknown origin.

The terms **heart failure (HF), congestive heart failure (CHF),** and

cardiomyopathy are often used interchangeably, but ought not to be. *Cardiomyopathy* is a disease that weakens heart muscle; *heart failure* is its most common manifestation, and *congestive heart failure* occurs when ongoing heart failure leads to a buildup of fluid that congests the body. More important than knowing the terminology is understanding that heart failure can involve a malfunction of either the heart's ability to contract and pump blood, or expand and be refilled with blood. (For basics about heart anatomy and mechanics, log on to the American Heart Association Web site: www.americanheart.org.) In case you don't have Internet access, I'll go over some details here.

LEFT-SIDED HEART FAILURE

In a healthy cardiovascular system, oxygen-rich blood rushes from the lungs into the upper left chamber of the heart, known as the left atrium. The blood then flows into the left ventricle, which contracts and pumps the blood toward the rest of the body. (The rhythmic, repetitive contraction of the heart's chambers is sometimes referred to as *systole;* the expansion of the chambers when they fill with blood is known as *diastole.*)

When the ventricles become enlarged due to the progression of heart failure, muscle fibers stretch and the heart loses its strength. This causes *systolic dysfunction,* a weakening of the heart's pumping action, which accounts for the lowered ejection fraction seen in this form of the disease. The majority of HF patients younger than sixty-five suffer from systolic dysfunction.

If the heart muscle gets too thick and stiff, it is unable to expand to its former capacity and not enough blood enters the ventricles. This condition is called *diastolic dysfunction,* and it accounts for most HF problems in elderly patients. Interestingly, the prognosis is better if you've got diastolic rather than systolic dysfunction.

When your heart doesn't pump properly for a long time, it could lead to *congestive heart failure (CHF).* If you've been diagnosed with CHF, it means your heart's decreased pumping ability has caused fluids to accumulate in your body. This happens because the ventricles cannot pump out all the blood that entered them, and the incoming blood adds yet more which the ventricles are incapable of dispatching. The blood begins to back up into the lungs. This is when congestion occurs: you begin to have shortness of breath (dyspnea) or swelling in the legs and feet (edema). In advanced stages, fluid accumulates in the abdominal cavity (ascites), causing the belly to swell.

If you have left-sided heart failure, you're likely to suffer from fatigue and shortness of breath (whether you're active or resting), and to cough up blood-tinged sputum. Lying flat may also pose a problem and cause you to wake up coughing during the night due to shortness of breath (paroxysmal nocturnal dyspnea, or PND). If you have CHF, you might have to prop yourself up with pillows in order to sleep. Physicians sometimes use the number of pillows a patient needs to gauge the severity of the CHF. Sometimes pillows aren't enough; one well-known CHF patient, Franklin Delano Roosevelt, had to sleep in a chair.

RIGHT-SIDED HEART FAILURE

When the heart's left side fails to do its job, it often means trouble for the right side as well. In fact, right-sided heart failure is most often caused by left-sided failure.

Here's why. The upper right chamber of the heart, or right atrium, receives oxygen-depleted blood as it returns from nourishing the rest of the body. The blood flows from the right atrium down to the right ventricle, which then pumps it into the lungs to be replenished with oxygen. Right-sided or right-ventricular heart failure usually occurs when fluid accumulated in the lungs due to left-ventricle dysfunction backs up and damages the right side of the heart. When the right side loses its pumping power, blood backs up in the veins, causing swelling in the legs and ankles.

With all this excess fluid trapped in the body, HF patients often feel an urge to urinate, especially at night. Fluid buildup overloads the kidneys, limiting their ability to dispose of salt (sodium chloride) and water. If left untreated, this may lead to kidney failure. Obviously, if your body is retaining fluid, you should see a physician and have it treated. It's worth the effort: once this aspect of heart failure is treated, the kidneys typically return to normal.

Other symptoms of congestive heart failure include:

- Weight gain due to accumulated fluid.
- Chest pain.
- Increased fatigue. Because the heart cannot pump an adequate amount of blood, the body diverts blood from large muscles and redirects it to vital organs.
- Diminished appetite or a feeling of indigestion due to insufficient blood in the digestive system.

- Swollen neck veins.
- Cold, clammy skin.
- Rapid or irregular pulse due to the heart having to work harder. It may also include increased ventricular tachycardia, an abnormally high ventricular rhythm which may worsen until it becomes ventricular fibrillation, a potentially fatal, unregulated series of very rapid contractions.
- Restlessness, confusion, and diminishment of attention span and memory due to weakened blood flow to the brain or to changes in blood chemistry, often involving substances such as salt.
- Bluish tinge to the skin due to diminished oxygen supply.
- Inability to shake a cold or other minor illnesses.

Although the symptoms sound grave, congestive heart failure typically progresses slowly and allows many patients to enjoy active, even adventurous lives. The New York Heart Association describes four categories of CHF, classified by the degree to which symptoms impair a patient's ability to complete daily activities:

- **Class I:** Patients can go about ordinary physical activities without symptoms.
- **Class II:** Patients suffer from slight limitations; some activities, such as walking up a hill, cause shortness of breath.
- **Class III:** Patients report marked limitations and symptoms occur with little exertion; walking on a level surface can cause shortness of breath.
- **Class IV:** Patients report severe limitations; they may experience breathlessness while at rest.

Heart failure is a serious condition, and it wears people down. Patients who have it show higher levels of depression, hostility, and anxiety than those with other forms of heart illness. They also endure more interruptions to their work schedules and must limit their daily activities more stringently. So, you might ask, "Can I live with this condition and still have a life, and maybe even be *happy?*"

The answer is a resounding *yes!* Some of my patients have other illnesses along with heart failure, have endured medical setbacks, and still are the epitome of resilience: their will to thrive prevails over hard times, and they maintain a hopeful attitude that enables them to see the richness and possibility of life.

This is not let's-think-happy-thoughts-and-feel-better pseudopsychology; it's the truth: **if you have heart failure, the way you and your family cope with it could influence your fate more decisively than anything else.**

HEART FAILURE CLINICS

These relatively new programs assemble physicians, nurses, and other practitioners who have devoted their careers to helping heart failure patients stay healthy and manage the disease. When you visit such a clinic regularly, people check to make sure you're taking your medications properly and maintaining a healthy weight. They look for signs that your condition might be worsening, and immediately treat the underlying problem. Some clinics have doctors and nurses who make house calls, and a phone number you can call for help with questions or problems.

These programs are still too new to offer conclusive data on their effectiveness, but so far they seem to lower the frequency, severity, and duration of their participants' hospital stays, as well as keep a watchful eye on their symptoms so they may be treated promptly. Heart failure clinics will likely become the mainstay of care for this condition in the near future.

Research backs me up. When heart failure patients participate in programs that teach them how to cope, their lives get better even though the disease remains. *You have the power to do this:* exercising, learning how to manage stress, going for cognitive-behavioral therapy, taking biofeedback relaxation training, and enrolling in a heart failure clinic are things you can do, and all have been shown to diminish anxiety and depression in patients with heart failure, as well as improve the quality of their lives.[8]

WEIGHING WHAT YOU ACHIEVE
AGAINST WHAT YOU EXPECT

In the late 1800s, psychologist William James theorized that contentment and self-esteem are determined by the ratio between what we achieve and what we expect. Each of us knows this on some level: if you're always expecting perfect family harmony, you probably won't be content unless you wake up living with Ward and June Cleaver and the boys. On the other hand, if you have realistic notions about marital and family life, you've got a better shot at enjoying true contentment with the people dearest to you.

The psychology of living well with heart failure isn't so different: you must adjust your expectations to conform to what you can realistically achieve and celebrate your every whisper, shadow, and centimeter of success. If you don't, you'll be disappointed by your physical limitations and perceived lack of progress and render yourself vulnerable to frustration and despair.

You and your family are more likely to meet this challenge if you:

1. Learn about what heart failure is (and isn't).
2. Use common-sense strategies for managing your emotions, daily activities, and health behaviors.
3. Familiarize yourselves with the medications the patient must take to control the disease.
4. Stay abreast of the latest medical advances in treating the disease so you can make intelligent and well-informed decisions about your care.

You already know what heart failure is, so let's move on to number 2—your emotions and your way of life.

2. Use Common-sense Strategies for Managing Your Emotions, Daily Activities, and Health Behaviors.

First and absolutely foremost: don't try to do this alone. Managing heart failure is not something you should approach in isolation, however independent and disciplined you are. A sturdy self-concept and capacity for hard work are not all you need to win this war.

To reinforce and defend your state of mind, you need support from your friends, your family, and especially your life partner. Don't underestimate the impact of soulful energy—if you let it surround you, it can pull you to safety as well as any life preserver. James C. Coyne and his colleagues at the University of Pennsylvania followed 139 men and 50 women with congestive heart failure as well as their partners and found that *patients who got along well with their mates were more likely to be alive after four years than those in more contentious partnerships.* They also found that an agreeable primary relationship improved survival rates of patients with less severe disease. In Coyne's words, "How well a couple is working together predicts which patients with chronic heart failure will be alive in four years." [9] You can't get much clearer—or unequivocal—than that.

If you have heart failure, live alone, and don't have a network of friends, you must put energy into seeking companionship. You *must* battle the temptation to become a hermit; you must not surrender to grief. Learning you have an incurable illness (manageable, but incurable) may stoke flames of denial, desperation, and rage in your breast. Even patients who have coped well with a variety of diagnoses often have difficulty bouncing back when heart failure darkens the mix.

Battle any forces that threaten to bog you down in depression and grief. Cardiologist Marc Silver asserts, "[O]ptimistic heart failure patients do far better than pessimistic ones. . . . You must believe in the possibility of improvement. . . . Individuals with heart failure don't improve unless they see the possibility of improvement."[10]

Choose hope; reject despair. Work at accepting that which you cannot change, and changing what you can. Cherish your family and friends, and nurture your relationships. Keep your life up and running, even if walking is all you can manage. Heart failure patients who have poor quality of life are more likely to end up back in the hospital, and are also more likely to die.

This is especially true for women. As I mentioned earlier, female heart patients usually receive less physical and emotional support when coming home from the hospital than men do; this can have catastrophic consequences for women with HF. In the year following a hospital stay, female HF patients are more likely than male patients to suffer another, possibly fatal, cardiac event.[11] We also know that supportive relationships are equal opportunity lifesavers: both male and female CHF patients who are socially isolated are more likely to die than their more outgoing brothers and sisters.[12]

So don't keep people at arm's length; pull them toward you. If you live alone (and even if you don't), I recommend that you join a cardiac rehabilitation program, regularly visit an HF clinic, or join an HF support group, which typically involves family members as well as patients. The medical care and guidance these programs provide will monitor your symptoms and keep them in check, and the encouragement and reassurance will reinforce your resolve to stick to your heart-healthy habits. (See Resources for information about support programs.)

Tips for Changing Your Activities and Health Behaviors

More than any other cardiac condition, heart failure requires diligent, daily management of health behaviors. This illness provides an immediate reflection of how you treat your body—what you eat and drink, whether you exert yourself too much or not enough, how long you sit or stand.

If you've committed to your new normal, on the other hand, and manage your health behaviors well, your symptoms may quickly subside, and you may actually slow the progression of the disease.

Here are some tips on how to manage ten areas of crucial importance if you have heart failure: **stress, sleep, smoking, salt, medication, alcohol, fluids, caffeine, weight,** and **activities.** Whereas many of them apply to all heart patients, those with HF must take them particularly seriously.

STRESS

Heart failure patients live in a constant biological state of stress and must learn to manage it. As the disease progresses and heart damage increases, the body senses danger and releases stress hormones, norepinephrine chief among them, that activate the fight-or-flight response. Unfortunately, this simply makes things worse. Blood vessels constrict and prompt the fatigued (and probably enlarged) heart to pump faster and work harder, causing it to fail further.

As you develop strategies for coping with HF, be aware that you are living with elevated stress levels all the time. (See Chapter 6 for tips on how to manage stress.)

SLEEP

Sleep deprivation makes everything worse. Even healthy young people who become sleep-deprived show signs of coping poorly. Sleep deprivation can lead to irritability and depression, memory and concentration problems, and various body aches and pains, even if you don't have heart failure. Add to this the coughing caused by fluid backing up into the lungs, frequent middle-of-the-night urination due to excess fluid pooling in the bladder and the use of diuretics, and the effects of other medications, and it's no wonder that it's hard to cope if you're a heart failure patient who is also exhausted.

Fortunately, help is available. Look back at Chapter 6 for suggestions on how to create an environment that's conducive to sleep. And for information about diuretics and how to deal with them, see p. 212.

Finally, even on your worst days, it's important to spend a minimum of several hours upright and moving around, no matter how tired you feel. Ask family members and friends to drag you out for a short walk, or take you to the library, or engage you in short bouts of activity several times each day.

Smoking

If you smoke, quit. Fluids have already claimed valuable air rights in your lungs and diminished their capacity. Don't make matters worse by smoking.

Salt

Closely monitor your intake of salt (aka sodium chloride, or simply sodium) and stick to a low-sodium diet. The average American ingests about 4,000 milligrams, or 4 grams, of salt each day. Most HF patients are warned against ingesting more than 2,000 milligrams, or 2 grams, a day. Your doctor may recommend that you use even less.

Many people find it difficult to give up salt. Most of us have been consuming high-sodium foods our entire lives, and our taste buds clamor for them. Chips, pretzels, fast foods, deli meats, hot dogs, cheese—it seems that everything we love to eat is loaded with salt.

Give yourself time. The taste for salt is an acquired one. Your tongue will grow satisfied with pinches rather than oceans of salt, and you *will* enjoy food again—I guarantee it. Remind yourself that every low-salt mouthful brings you one bite closer to the meal you're waiting for—the one that actually tastes better *without* salt. By cutting down on your sodium intake, you'll wean yourself away from salt and actually start to dislike it. It's hard to do at first, but it will make an enormous difference in how effectively you manage this disease.

Start the process by learning the salt content of various foods. What you discover might surprise you. Here are some tips to help you to shake the salt habit: [13]

- **Read labels.** If a food has a label, the amount of sodium it contains will be on it. Don't be lulled into a false sense of security by salt substitutes, which are typically potassium rather than sodium salts. **High levels of potassium salts can be dangerous, so avoid those as well.**
- Banish the saltshaker from the table.
- When you cook, use half as much salt as the recipe calls for.
- Find a low-salt cookbook. There are hundreds out there.
- Avoid high-salt items such as:
  - MSG (monosodium glutamate), a flavor-enhancing ingredient sometimes used in Chinese cooking.
  - Soy sauce.
  - Catsup (aka ketchup), no matter what color it is.

- Baking soda (at least in food; feel free to use it on the laundry).
- Canned soups, broths, and bouillon.
- Snack foods. Read their labels very carefully. There are very good reduced-salt, low-salt, and even no-salt crackers, pretzels, and other snacks. Pop your own popcorn and don't add salt. (If you're in the market for a popper, get the kind that uses hot air—it works without oil and requires little clean-up.)
- Processed foods ("American cheese *food,*" for example), canned foods, and prepared sauces and salad dressings.
- Substitute herbs for salt. You'll find many you like.
- Eat at home as much as possible. When you dine in a restaurant, ask the server to point out low-sodium items. Ask that your food be cooked without added salt.
- If you use an antacid, choose one that's low in sodium.
- Salt substitutes may spice up your meals, but get your doctor's approval before you use them. Many contain potassium, and, as noted above, too much potassium can be dangerous.

MEDICATION

Take your medications exactly as prescribed. Even slight lapses can make big differences in fluid retention, heart rhythm control, and other important aspects of your prognosis and comfort. (I'll talk more about medication later in this chapter.)

ALCOHOL

Avoid alcohol; it can weaken heart muscle and lead to a condition called alcoholic cardiomyopathy. If you have alcoholic cardiomyopathy, you should quit drinking, period. If you have a different type of cardiomyopathy, it isn't clear whether or not you need to stop completely. However, since alcohol can cause heart muscle to deteriorate, all HF patients should refrain from drinking.

FLUIDS

Monitor your fluid intake. More than other heart patients, those with HF must control the amount of fluid they drink and keep it in the range of one to two quarts a day. Drinking too much of anything can cause a buildup of fluid in your body, which can complicate your condition. Your margin for error here is small: drinking as little as two cups over your allotted amount could increase your body weight by a pound. The frequent mistake HF patients make is forgetting that any food that either liquefies at room temperature or can be poured is considered a fluid. That means that foods such as Jell-O and ice cream count as fluids and can make you overflow your limit if you eat them thinking they're solids.

Here's a technique to help you keep track of your fluid intake: first thing each morning, fill a pitcher with an amount of water equal to your daily fluid allowance. Every time you sip a beverage or eat a food that counts as a fluid, pour the corresponding amount of water out of the pitcher. By glancing at the pitcher, you'll be reminded of how much fluid remains in your allowance for the day.

CAFFEINE

Avoid caffeine and other substances that stimulate the heart. Stimulants make your heart beat more rapidly, can cause heart rhythm irregularities, and increase the amount of oxygen your heart needs. Your heart is already overworked; don't burden it unnecessarily. Coffee, tea, colas and other soft drinks, and chocolate all contain caffeine.

WEIGHT

Weigh yourself every day. A sudden weight gain may signal that you're retaining fluid, even if you feel well. If you put on more than three pounds in a day or five pounds in a week, you probably need to adjust something. Call your doctor.

ACTIVITIES

Find the right balance between rest and activity. This is a day-to-day proposition for many HF patients. As I mentioned earlier, it is crucial that you be upright and moving about for at least part of the day, even if your heart failure is at an advanced stage. On the other hand, it is essential that you get enough rest and put your feet up whenever you can to reduce ankle swelling. The key is to be realistic when planning your activities, and to know your limitations.

- **Put exercise into perspective.** Remember that, when you are an HF patient, your heart is always overworked, even when you're sleeping. Your job is to find an activity level that will give you the benefits of exercising without further burdening your heart. Before starting an exercise program, it is important that you get advice from your physician. Find out *how long, how hard,* and *how often* you should exercise, and remember these rules:

- Start slowly and build up gradually.

- Exercises that work the large leg muscles create less immediate cardiac strain than those that use the arms.

- Stop exercising *immediately* if you are dizzy, have chest pain, or become shorter of breath than usual.

- The "no pain, no gain" anthem is sheer foolishness that can be dangerous to your health. If you are too short of breath to carry on a conversation while you are exercising, slow down or stop.

- **Learn to work smarter.** Conserve your energy so you have enough to do the things you have to do and want to do. Here are some tips:

  - Avoid rushing. Plan ahead, giving yourself enough time to get where you need to go and accomplish what needs to be done.

  - Approach tasks at a steady pace.

  - Remember that standing takes more energy than sitting. Whenever possible, pull up a chair.

  - Rest for at least thirty minutes after a meal before embarking on a task. When you work on a full stomach, your heart needs more oxygen, and will work harder to get it.

  - Avoid working in extreme heat (above 80° Fahrenheit, 27° Centigrade) or cold (below 20° Fahrenheit, −7° Centigrade).

  - Plan your activities so they are spread throughout the day.

  - Delegate tasks to others whenever you can, and hire people to do enervating chores.

  - Get enough sleep. This means scheduling an afternoon nap if you're planning to stay up late.

  - Rest between tasks. Many patients find it helpful to take several twenty- or thirty-minute breaks each day and to rest for ten to fifteen minutes whenever they get tired, even if they're in the midst of a task.

  - Before starting a task or project, ask yourself two questions:

    1. Is it important that I do this now? If not, when is another time I might do it?

    2. How can I make this easier on myself?

       - Should I get help?

       - Can I break this task into smaller, more manageable steps?

       - What can I do to increase my comfort while I accomplish this task?

  - Use common sense: activities that require you to push or pull burn more energy; upper-body activities place more demands on your heart. After a setback, increase your activities gradually. For instance, if you end up in bed with an upper respiratory infection or in the hospital for a few days because of some worrisome symptoms, take it easy when you resume your daily routine.

- Remember: small changes can make big differences in your recovery. For example, if a frequent need to urinate requires that your life revolve around the availability of a bathroom ask your doctor if you can take your diuretic at a different time of day. It's a small adjustment but one that could greatly expand the scope of your activity.

3. FAMILIARIZE YOURSELF WITH THE MEDICATIONS YOU *MUST* TAKE TO CONTROL THE DISEASE.

In addition to understanding the nature of heart failure and making a commitment to taking care of yourself, you must also have a grasp of the medications that enable you to live well with this disease. A typical regimen includes multiple medications from several categories. I'll explain these in the pages that follow. (See the Appendix for lists of medications by category.)

Vasodilators: Angiotensin-Converting Enzyme (ACE) Inhibitors and Others

Vasodilators (substances that dilate, or expand, blood vessels) are the cornerstone of drug therapy for heart failure. ACE inhibitors boost HF patients' stamina for everyday activities and exercise, modulate their symptoms, and help them live longer, increasing survival rates by as much as 40 percent.

Angiotensin is a hormone secreted by the kidneys that causes small arteries to constrict. When this happens, less blood can pass through the vessels, blood pressure goes up, and the heart works harder to keep things moving. By blocking angiotensin, ACE inhibitors help keep arteries dilated so blood can flow more freely. Side effects may include skin rash, cough, lowered blood pressure, and changed perceptions of the taste of food.

Two other vasodilators favored by physicians are calcium channel blockers and nitrates. Calcium channel blockers are occasionally prescribed for use with beta-blockers and ACE inhibitors to lighten the heart's workload.

Nitrates are also popular vasodilators, but remember:

If you are taking nitrates, beware of interactions between these medications with others such as Viagra, which may cause serious drops in blood pressure.

For information about interactions between nitrates and other drugs, see Chapter 9.

Diuretics

Commonly known as water pills, diuretics are standard therapy for heart failure patients. They expedite the processing of excess fluid through the kidneys and result in more frequent urination.

Diuretics are powerful drugs. They may cause dehydration and lower the concentration of electrolytes in the body, which may prompt irregular heartbeats and impaired heart function. (Electrolytes are charged particles of salts such as sodium, potassium, or magnesium, which dissolve in the body's fluids. The body must maintain the concentration of electrolytes to function properly.) Diuretics can also drain you of calcium, which may lead to deposits of uric acid and a painful attack of gout.

If you don't use diuretics properly, your blood pressure may dip dangerously low; you might also develop kidney problems. Be sure to keep your physician posted about your use of diuretics.

Diuretics will also have you running to the bathroom more often. This can be inconvenient, especially when you're traveling, going out for the evening, or planning on being away from modern plumbing for any amount of time. As a result, some patients stop taking their diuretics, which is usually a mistake. Instead, as mentioned earlier, ask your physician for advice on changing the time you take the diuretic.

Digoxin (Lanoxin, Digitalis)

In use since the eighteenth century, this medication has made a comeback in recent years. It strengthens the heart's pumping action and increases the left ventricular ejection fraction. It is administered to slow the heartbeat in cases of atrial fibrillation. Digoxin is the medication of choice for someone whose heart pumps too weakly (a systolic problem), but not useful for someone whose heart has trouble relaxing or expanding (a diastolic problem).

If you take digoxin, your condition must be closely monitored, especially if you also are taking a diuretic or the powerful anti-arrhythmic amiodarone (marketed as Cordarone and Pacerone). The effects of digoxin may be drastically altered by interactions with other drugs and even by some foods.

Beta-Blockers

Beta-blockers check the effects of adrenaline on the body, slowing the heart and lightening its load. Beta-blockers also lower blood pressure. They are often used in conjunction with ACE inhibitors and diuretics.

Coumadin

Patients with heart failure, damaged heart valves, or irregular heartbeat (especially atrial fibrillation, an abnormally rapid contraction of the ventricles) are at risk of forming blood clots in the heart. If these embolize, or break off, they can travel to other parts of the body and cause serious problems, especially in the lungs and the brain. To prevent this, your physician may prescribe a blood thinner known as Coumadin (warfarin sodium), which reduces the blood's ability to clot. Coumadin's effectiveness is affected by foods containing vitamin K and many common medications such as aspirin, antihistamines, and birth control pills. If you take Coumadin, it is crucial that you have your blood checked regularly to assure that your prothrombin time ("pro-time," for short)—the number of seconds needed for your blood to clot—is still low enough to allow your blood to clot before you lose too much of it.

4. STAY ABREAST OF THE LATEST MEDICAL ADVANCES IN TREATING THE DISEASE SO YOU CAN MAKE INTELLIGENT, WELL-INFORMED DECISIONS ABOUT YOUR CARE.

This is the final component of living well with heart failure. We have known for many years that some HF cases can be improved through surgery: repairing or replacing damaged valves, a bypass, or correcting congenital defects. Because heart failure is a growing public health threat, researchers are forging ahead in the field and making rapid progress. New developments crop up all the time, and you can find out about them if you make the effort. I have heard heart failure specialists complain that their colleagues sometimes know less about the disease than their patients! Knowing your options will help you get the most out of your consultations with physicians and other medical personnel.

The way to do this is to immerse yourself in information from any and all sources: newspapers, magazines, books, radio, television, and the Internet are all bursting with it. By aggressively seeking and sharing information related to heart-healthy living, you establish yourself in your physicians' eyes as a well-informed, educated patient who will settle for nothing less than the finest medical care.

Here are a few procedures worth knowing about:

Cardiac Resynchronization Therapy (Biventricular Pacing)

Pacemakers prevent the heart from beating too slowly (for more on this and automatic implantable cardioverter defibrillators, or ICDs, see Chapter 12). While this isn't the primary problem facing heart failure patients, there is substantial evidence that some people with severe HF or conduction disorders, especially those with cardiomyopathy, may benefit from dual-chamber pacemakers that resynchronize the heart's activity.

About a third of HF patients (and some heart patients without HF) have an abnormality in the heart's electrical system called a bundle branch block disturbance that results in the two ventricles beating out of phase and throwing heart coordination out of synch. By activating both ventricles simultaneously, cardiac resynchronization improves the mechanical efficiency of the heart, leading to a decrease in the frequency of ventricular arrhythmias and improvements in blood pressure, exercise capacity, and overall quality of life.[14]

As of August 2002, two biventricular pacing devices had been approved by the FDA: Guidant's Contac CD (a combination cardiac resynchronization device and implantable defibrillator), and Medtronic's InSync device. The InSync device has gotten a lot of publicity lately, thanks to the Multicenter InSync Randomized Clinical Evaluation, or MIRACLE trial, which was designed to more definitively measure the effectiveness and safety of cardiac resynchronization therapy (CRT) for treating heart failure.[15] The study involved five hundred patients with advanced congestive heart failure and found that, after six months, those who had received the InSync device had markedly improved quality of life, exercise stamina, and ability to perform everyday tasks, and required hospitalization only half as often as those who did not receive the device. And when patients with the device did enter the hospital, they remained there for a briefer period than patients without it; as a group, they spent one quarter as many days in the hospital as the control group. A year after the study ended, a follow-up survey indicated the results were holding fast.[16] This study, along with others, provides us with data on more than two thousand patients, suggesting that cardiac resynchronization therapy helps some people live longer and more happily with fewer medical complications.

Cardiac resynchronization therapy is the first nondrug medical treatment to improve the lives of HF patients so vastly, and offers them a hopeful future where there had been little to look forward to. The devices are costly and cardiologists must receive special training to implant them, but more and more physicians and facilities are qualifying to perform the procedure.

As this is a relatively new therapy, it may not be the first thing your doctor thinks of when contemplating your treatment. Assert yourself: speak up and ask if cardiac resynchronization might be a viable option for you. And remember—if a heart attack caused your heart failure, you're probably already a candidate for an implantable cardiac device. Be sure to ask your physician about one of these newer, combination-type devices.[17]

Heart Transplant

When enough of a person's heart muscle is damaged, he or she may teeter on the brink of death while the rest of the body is still in relatively good condition. This often happens when someone has an advanced case of heart failure, and it is then that heart transplantation becomes a consideration.

When I started working with cardiac patients, heart transplants were relatively rare, and people who had them faced dire consequences—lives fraught with such dread of rejection and infection of the new organ that they were reduced to living in what amounted to isolation. Today, however, new antibiotics and immunosuppressant drugs (substances that suppress the immune system's rejection of an implanted organ) have revolutionized a transplant patient's potential to survive beyond the sterile confines of the operating room. Eighty-five percent of transplant patients now live longer than a year after the surgery, and 65 percent survive for at least five years.

About forty thousand Americans need new hearts, but so few (about two thousand) are donated each year that priority is given to those patients who will live only a few more months unless they get a new one. To remedy this shortfall, scientists are focusing on xenotransplantation, implanting an animal heart (usually that of a pig or baboon) in a human.

Left Ventricular Assist Device (LVAD)

For a person awaiting a heart transplant, a left ventricular assist device, or LVAD, is a temporary lifesaver. Once it is implanted in the chest and connected to the patient's heart, the LVAD takes over the left ventricle's pumping action. Some people who have used the LVAD for a few months found it strengthened their own heart's ventricles. And some patients can even be weaned from the LVAD and no longer require a new heart.

In June 2003, *The New York Times* published a riveting story about Megan Ivers, a University of Minnesota freshman who almost died when a virus attacked her heart. Her one hope was an LVAD, which was implanted in her chest to keep her alive while she awaited a transplant. Less than three months later, doctors removed the device and Megan's heart continued to beat strongly on its own.[18]

LVADs have been used since 1998 to keep transplant patients alive until donor hearts become available. The Food and Drug Administration has approved several LVADs for use as interim implants; some are designed for use in-hospital while the patient awaits transplantation surgery; others are portable and allow patients to return home while they wait.

But LVADs are becoming much more common. Late in 2002, the FDA approved Thoratec's HeartMate device for use as a *permanent* implant, a new application cardiologists are calling "destination therapy." A recent study found that LVADs kept dying heart patients alive. But the pumps are far from flawless; they tend to break, and some patients who receive them get fatal injections. And at a price of $65,000 for the device and about $100,000 to implant it, the question arises as to which patients should get them and who should pay.

Implantable Hemodynamic Monitoring Device

Scientists are investigating this new machine, which could revolutionize treatment of heart failure patients by enabling physicians to check on their progress while the patients are at home. The device employs a sensor, activated either automatically or by the patient, that picks up and records data about the patient's bodily processes—heart rate, blood pressure, and a variety of others. The data are then downloaded from the patient's home via a remote monitor and transmitted to the physician's office via the Internet. The physician can read the information, interpret it, and advise the patient on how to remedy a problem without the patient ever having to leave the house. This device will enable a physician to diagnose and correct a medical problem before it evolves into a crisis, and confer greater efficiency on long-term medical care for HF patients.

Artificial Heart

Scientists have been working feverishly since 1982 to perfect a fully implantable, self-contained artificial heart, and are getting closer all the time. Their most recent effort is the AbioCor (pronounced AB-ee-o-kor)

Implantable Replacement Heart, made by Abiomed, Inc., which weighs two pounds and is about the size of a grapefruit.

A patient who receives an artificial heart gets a lot more than that: an internal coil, a controller, and a backup battery are all implanted along with the heart. Then there's the peripheral equipment, including special batteries, a power driver, and a transfer coil. The technology is still far from ideal, but it's getting there; a self-contained, permanent artificial heart will likely be perfected by 2010.

New Surgical Developments

Scientists are also developing new surgical options, two promising examples of which are the Batista procedure and dynamic cardiomyoplasty.

In the Batista procedure, named for the man who invented it, a surgeon carves away excess tissue from a heart whose muscle has grown too large to function efficiently. In dynamic cardiomyoplasty, a surgeon removes a section of muscle from the patient's back, wraps it around the damaged heart, and implants a special pacemaker that stimulates the wrap to contract, bolstering the heart's own contractions.

Both these surgeries are new and have not yet been widely utilized and tested. But more of them are done each day, and more data about them will soon become available.

WHEN TO CALL THE DOCTOR

How do you know when a symptom is worrisome enough to warrant a call to the doctor? You won't hasten your recovery if you're alarmed by every twinge and hiccup. On the other hand, waiting too long to get medical care might cause unnecessary complications and even death. If you have heart failure, you can manage the disease if you **see a doctor promptly when you need to, and you need to if:**

- You have pain or tightness in your chest.
- Your breathing problems have gotten noticeably worse.
- You are unusually tired or weak most of the time.
- Your feet, legs, or stomach tend to swell.
- You have a cough that will not go away.
- You are coughing up blood-tinged sputum.

- You have gained three pounds or more within the last two days.
- You must prop yourself up with more and more pillows in order to sleep.
- You are waking up at night gasping for breath.
- You are getting up more frequently at night to urinate.
- You are experiencing dizziness worse than the mild variety that sometimes occurs when you stand up too quickly.
- Your heart is beating irregularly, or you are having palpitations.
- You lose consciousness.

A heart failure patient personifies paradox: he or she persists at living, beat by beat, to the rhythm of a damaged heart. I have witnessed these valiant men and women wage campaigns against an illness whose prognosis is never rosy and learned much about courage from them and their families.

You too can thrive with this condition if you accept the reality of your mortality and draw from it not despair but the determination to cherish every moment you've been granted. That is, when you think about it, all any of us has to live for.

Chapter Twelve

LIVING WELL WITH AN IMPLANTABLE CARDIOVERTER DEFIBRILLATOR (ICD)

Ventricular tachycardia, the condition I developed

during surgery, has no ambiguity. It simply results in

sudden cardiac death, unless you have an ICD.

—DEBORAH DAW HEFFERNAN [1]

The implantable cardioverter defibrillator, or ICD, is a small device with a big name and enormous implications for heart patients. Deborah Daw Heffernan is one of them: athletic, fit, and health-conscious, she was nearly killed by a heart attack at the age of forty-four. Today she travels and speaks publicly about heart disease with an ICD implanted in her chest.

Approved by the Food and Drug Administration in 1985, ICDs ushered in a new era in the treatment of life-threatening arrhythmias. Approximately 125,000 people with heart rhythm disturbances currently have ICDs, and they're about to have company: according to a study published in *The New England Journal of Medicine* in 2002,[2] this device can also help a much larger group of patients—those who have serious heart attack damage and are at risk for an arrhythmia but have yet to experience one. About 4 million Americans are in this category, with 400,000 more joining each year.

This broadening of the ICD's applicability has flung it onto the front pages of national newspapers in stories that discuss, among other things, the costs involved ($20,000 for the device, $10,000 for the surgery to implant it) and the tribulations of living with an electronic shock dispenser in your chest. But contrary to some quotes from patients about living with the misery of sporadic shocks,[3] the vast majority of ICD recipients say the device has improved their lives, that they would recommend it to anyone who needed it, and they would do it all over again if they had to reconsider the decision.[4]

ICDs save lives. A 1996 study of the effectiveness of ICDs versus drugs at controlling chronic arrhythmias found that half as many ICD patients died as those who received medication alone.[5] Another study monitored the progress of arrhythmia patients for three years and reported in 1998 that the death rate for ICD recipients was one third lower than that of patients who received standard medication treatment.[6] The most recent research with heart attack survivors in danger of developing arrhythmias is compelling. A group of these patients with extremely low ventricular ejection fractions were given ICDs as a precaution. Compared to patients who received only medication, those with defibrillators were one third as likely to die.[7] And in the study of New York–area heart patients who suffered dangerous arrythmias after the September 11 terrorist attacks, none of them had a heart attack or died: all 200 participants had ICDs.[8]

ICDS IMPROVE FAMILY LIFE, TOO

More good news about living with an ICD comes from research I conducted with the University of Florida's Samuel F. Sears, Ph.D., an internationally recognized expert on the psychology of living with implanted cardiac devices. In 1999, Sam and I led a team that conducted the largest survey ever taken of ICD recipients. We questioned 450 patients, 347 husbands, wives, and life partners, 103 electrophysiologists (cardiologists who specialize in implanting ICDs and interpreting the data they record), and 157 nurses about their experiences living with and treating people with ICDs.

And we got great news: ICD patients said that, unequivocally, the device had vastly improved their lives. After they received their ICDs:

- Ninety-one percent said the quality of their lives was just as good or better than before.
- Ninety-eight percent said their families were getting along better.
- Eighty-five percent said their emotional well-being had improved.[9]

But ICD patients and their family members must make significant adjustments, and not many people understand enough about the device to offer them the help they need. In fact, not many people even knew what an implantable defibrillator was until Vice President Dick Cheney got one. And it's not as if it's a familiar term even now; at one of my lectures, a woman described what happened when she told her sister she was getting an ICD: "Why do you need one?" asked her sister. "I thought you already had a hysterectomy!"

There's a big difference between an ICD and IUD, and that's putting it mildly.

WHAT IS THIS THING, AND WHY DO I NEED IT?

Roughly the size of three silver dollars and weighing less than a pound, an ICD is a small computer programmed to monitor and record heart activity, and deliver an electrical shock to correct any rhythm disturbances it detects. It is usually positioned just beneath the collarbone and contains wires, or leads, that issue from its center and are threaded into the heart, where they detect electrical impulses that have gone awry and caused an arrhythmia.

There are two basic kinds of arrhythmias: when the heart beats too quickly, or when it beats too slowly. A normal heartbeat ranges between 60 and 100 beats a minute, with most people coming in at about 72. When a heart beats over 100 times a minute, we say a person is suffering from tachycardia. With tachycardia, both the lower (ventrical) and upper (atrial) chambers can get out of rhythm, and these arrhythmias may either occur in a recognizable pattern or in a chaotic, unpredictable way. Fibrillation, a chaotic arrhythmia, is the most dangerous. At the other end of the scale is bradycardia, the term for when a person's heart beats too slowly, less than 60 beats per minute. When this happens, not enough blood flows to the body, causing a person to feel tired, short of breath, dizzy, and sometimes to lose consciousness.

Most people with bradycardia find relief with a pacemaker. Like an ICD, a pacemaker is a small computer programmed to monitor heart activity. It differs from an ICD in that it specializes in treating bradycardia, and emits short electrical impulses when the heart rate drops below a certain level. Patients say they usually don't feel any discomfort as a result of these impulses. And contrary to what you might have heard, pacemakers do not set off metal detectors at airports, nor are they affected by garage door openers, electric blankets, heating pads, or later-model microwave ovens (some early ones did interfere with pacemaker activity).

But some patients need more protection than a pacemaker can offer, and that's when an ICD saves lives—by diagnosing heart rhythms that are too rapid or too slow and delivering a shock (or series of shocks) to reset the pace. An ICD delivers several kinds of impulses, depending on what it detects:

- **Anti-tachycardia pacing:** delivers (usually painless) electrical impulses that interrupt an episode of arrhythmia and restore normal heart rhythm

221

- **Defibrillation:** delivers (usually perceptible, often uncomfortable, sometimes painful) high-level electrical shocks to correct serious arrhythmias, such as ventricular tachycardia or ventricular fibrillation

In the past, ICDs were reserved for patients with tachycardia, but newer models have been designed to treat bradycardia as well. These new devices act as combination ICDs and permanent pacemakers. We may also soon see implanted devices that automatically release antiarrhythmic and heart failure medications.

An ICD also performs another important function: it stores information about heart rhythms, so when you come in for your appointment, your physician can "interrogate" the device and get a complete beat-by-beat history of your heart's behaviors over the last several months. This interrogation also lets your physician check the ICD's battery level and lead system. (An ICD generator may last up to five years, depending on several factors, among them how many shocks it has delivered.)

And now you might not even have to leave the house: a recently unveiled generation of smart ICDs and pacemakers allows physicians to interrogate the devices electronically while patients remain at home (for information about similar technology for treating congestive heart failure—implantable hemodynamic monitoring devices, still in the trial stage—see Chapter 11).

One of these new ICDs is manufactured by Medtronic, which sponsors Care-Link, an Internet-based monitoring network. Patients who have the Medtronic device can transmit information stored on their ICDs by holding a small monitor up to their collarbones (or wherever the ICD is implanted). The monitor picks up the information and transfers it via telephone modem to the network's secure server, where it can then be accessed by doctors and nurses. They then check the condition of the device, making sure the battery is charged and the leads in place, and decide whether or not the patient must come in to the office for an examination. Insurance carriers as well as Medicare have agreed to pay for patient participation in this program in many states.

The CareLink site also contains a wealth of information to help patients and their families develop skills for coping with an ICD. So far, physicians and patients alike have given the site high marks, and I recommend it without reservation because it was designed by my good friend Dr. Sam Sears and me. (For more information about the CareLink program, log on to www.medtronic.com/newsroom/media_kits.html.)

These innovations aren't only for patients with ICDs—similar technology has been developed for home monitoring of pacemaker data.[10] In this case, the patient uses a monitor to transmit information from the pacemaker to a receiver in his or her home, which then sends the information to a computer service center. The center then issues a brief printed report that can be faxed to a physician if necessary.

DO YOU NEED AN ICD?

An ICD might be appropriate for you if you suffer from any of the following symptoms:

- If you experience syncope (loss of consciousness) due to unknown causes and accompanied by evidence of ventricular tachycardia (VT) or ventricular fibrillation (VF).
- If you've been taking medication but it isn't working, or you are not tolerating it well, or your physician deems it insufficient to control your heart rhythm problems.
- If you have a family history of life-threatening ventricular arrhythmias such as long-QT syndrome (a condition characterized by frequent fainting coupled with an extended interval between blood-pumping heartbeats) or hypertrophic cardiomyopathy (a congenital condition that causes the walls of the ventricles to thicken abnormally).
- If your ejection fraction is less than 30 percent; in other words, if your heart is able to pump out only a third or less of the blood inside it. A healthy heart pumps out with each beat at least half the blood it contains. Doctors use ejection fraction to assess the damage caused by a heart attack specifically and heart disease in general.

KNOW YOUR EJECTION FRACTION!

As a heart patient, you should be as aware of your ejection fraction as you are of your cholesterol level, blood pressure, and other risk factors. Why? Because if your ejection fraction is less than 30 percent, you may feel fine but still be at risk for developing a deadly arrhythmia.

The next time you see your doctor, ask for information about your ejection fraction.

SUDDEN CARDIAC ARREST

While most ICDs are prescribed for arrhythmia patients, doctors also recommend them for people suffering from a serious condition known as sudden cardiac arrest (SCA). Sudden cardiac arrest (sometimes referred to as sudden cardiac death, or SCD) is a face-off with death that comes without warning. Unlike a heart attack, which results when a blocked artery prevents blood and oxygen from reaching the heart, sudden cardiac arrest is usually the result of an electrical disturbance in a part of the heart that's already been damaged and scarred. According to Barry W. Ramo, M.D., a heart scar can create a situation "much like putting your finger in a light socket. It causes the heart muscle to quiver, and stop pumping blood to the body, and can result in death in a matter of minutes." [11]

Sudden cardiac arrest follows a fairly predictable pattern, and it's not a pretty one. A person, often thought to be in good health, suddenly collapses. The brain is deprived of oxygen, rendering him or her unconscious and gasping for air. At this point, the person may have a seizure and lose bladder control. If the person isn't resuscitated within four minutes, there will be permanent brain damage; delays of eight to ten minutes result in death.

Most often, ventricular fibrillation is the culprit. Patients with underlying coronary artery disease and ventricular problems with low ejection fraction are at higher risk for developing SCA than other heart patients. About one third of the 400,000 Americans stricken each year with sudden cardiac arrest now survive the initial collapse, with the majority of them going on to receive an ICD. [12] (These patients sometimes experience cognitive difficulties after their implantation surgery; for more on this, see p. 226.)

PSYCHOLOGICAL STRATEGIES FOR DEALING WITH AN ICD

Until very recently, anyone who received an ICD had lived for years with a deteriorating heart condition that resulted in life-threatening irregular heartbeats. It's no wonder, then, that many ICD patients struggle. After the device is implanted, most patients complain of increased fear and nervousness, and about a third suffer from anxiety disorders. These symptoms aren't unique to ICD recipients; any patient with an implanted medical device may fear it won't work properly, and no one with a chronic illness is a stranger to the specter of death. In addition, ICD patients grapple with the fear of pain, loss of control, and embarrassment associated with being zapped by an unanticipated electrical shock.

As if fear of getting shocked were not enough, the ICD patient has another worry: What if I *don't* get a shock when I need one? Many of my ICD patients have trouble trusting that their battery will stay charged and their leads are in place. It's little wonder that between a quarter and a third of ICD patients are depressed.[13]

Family members struggle as well. A year after surgery, some life partners of ICD patients are more anxious than the patients themselves.[14] They may feel depressed, helpless, and stressed, and it gets worse if the patient has another cardiac event.

Here are the top ten coping challenges ICD patients and their loved ones face, according to our survey:

- Worry (generalized anxiety)
- Fear of physical exertion
- Fear of receiving an ICD discharge or shock, or needing one and *not* receiving it
- Dealing with shocks when they occur
- Sexual issues
- Returning to work
- Managing stress
- Difficulty relaxing (see above)
- Money worries
- Depression

Most patients receive an ICD only after they've been battling heart illness for a long time. But the moment the device is implanted in their breasts, these men and women are beset by new physical and psychological forces they must divide and conquer.

"I FEEL VIOLATED!"

"I don't even like to take medication—now this *thing* is stuck in my body forever. I *hate* this feeling!" These words echo those I've heard from many people when they get the device, at least at first.

Accepting and embracing the ghostly and eternal presence of a machine in your body is a new psychology. Patients wonder: What is it going to feel like? What does it mean if my illness has come to this? If I do survive, will I ever be able to let someone see me with my shirt off? How will I look with this bulge in my chest?

When you get an ICD, it's normal for you and your loved ones to have at least some periods of worry and distress. Similar to other heart patients, people who receive ICDs or suffer from sudden cardiac arrest experience their worst anxiety, depression, anger, stress, and denial within six months of getting out of the hospital.

The first few months are the hardest. It's crucial for patients and the people who care about them to be available emotionally to one another—especially as compassionate listeners—during this trying time. Everyone will be wrestling with different emotions, and the patient will be contending with bewildering physical adjustments as well.

For six to eight weeks after receiving the implant, you're likely to have numerous physical symptoms including lack of energy, breathlessness, dizziness, and weakness. You may not have the strength to conduct even simple activities such as walking the dog or transferring the laundry from the washer to the dryer. Side effects of antiarrhythmic medications may leave you nauseated. You may gain weight or you may lose it. Your incision may hurt, and you may have trouble sleeping.

SUDDEN CARDIAC ARREST PATIENTS MAY HAVE ADDITIONAL DIFFICULTIES

Survivors of sudden cardiac arrest may experience changes in cognitive functioning, their ability to think clearly and organize information. Forgetfulness, reduced attention span, and impaired ability to concentrate or solve basic problems may cause a patient to become increasingly irritable, impatient, and depressed. Family members may find themselves growing ill-tempered, as well, especially if the patient is unaware of his or her diminished capacity or refuses to acknowledge it.

It is often difficult to tell whether these deficits are caused by the interruption of the brain's oxygen supply during the SCA collapse or by underlying cardiac illness, medication, or depression. And research hasn't exactly cleared things up. Some studies claim that about half of SCA survivors experience memory and concentration problems within a year or two of the collapse.[15] Other studies are more reassuring, stating that patients who are alert for twelve to seventy-two hours after resuscitation usually do well neurologically.[16]

If you have experienced an episode of sudden cardiac arrest, it is highly likely you will suffer at least some degree of cognitive impairment, especially in the early stages of your recovery (see Chapter 2). Yet despite the prevalence of cognitive problems in cases of sudden cardiac arrest, survivors receive neither routine neurological examination nor neuropsychological testing when they are discharged from the hospital.[17] If you or your loved one has this trouble, insist on a referral for a neuropsychological evaluation.

MOST ICD RECIPIENTS ADJUST WELL

Far and away, most patients overcome their early ICD jitters, and they do it pretty quickly. Between six and twelve months after receiving the device, more than 95 percent say that they have adjusted to it and that the adjustments they had to make were worth the effort.[18]

If you are like most ICD patients, any distress you feel about carrying this pager-sized computer in your chest will soon be overridden by the realization that your only other option may be death. Of course, your adjustment will be rockier if you encounter a cardiac setback. This is particularly the case if you've been receiving multiple painful shocks. Few studies have investigated long-term adjustment to living with an ICD. But Dr. Sears and his colleagues at the University of Florida recently reported that patients who had lived with an ICD for up to four years did experience gradual declines in their quality of life if they received multiple shocks, were highly anxious, and had poor social support.[19]

ALL ABOUT SHOCKS

"Now that I've got this thing, does it mean I'm going to get shocked?"

When I counsel ICD patients, I probably hear this question more than any other. While it's true that 50 to 60 percent of ICD patients do receive a shock within a year of getting the device, these figures are shrinking.

Here's why. First, many of these shocks are responses to false alarms—a result of the device getting fooled into thinking that a life-threatening arrhythmia is occurring when it actually isn't. If your ICD detects a ventricular arrhythmia—a dangerously abnormal heart rhythm in the lower chambers of your heart—it will institute a series of therapies to correct the problem. These therapies sometimes include an uncomfortable or painful shock.

Occasionally, the *upper* chambers of the heart experience a supraventricular arrhythmia; in other words, their rhythm is disturbed—a momentary and, in most cases, non-life-threatening event. But these flutters in the upper chamber sometimes cause the ventricle beneath it to speed up a bit, just enough to fool the ICD into doing its job. The device fires and sends a substantial shock to the heart, which was never in any real danger.

As ICD technology improves (and it does every day), these inappropriate shocks will become increasingly rare. Some patients are already equipped with smarter ICDs that monitor both heart chambers; these patients are enduring far fewer inappropriate shocks.

The second reason fewer ICD patients are receiving unnecessary shocks is that, as mentioned earlier, many of them are using the devices as a precaution against arrhythmias they don't yet have. Since their hearts suffer fewer rhythm disturbances, they receive fewer shocks.

At this point, ICD patients receive an average of two shocks per year.[20] You're more likely to receive a shock if your ejection fraction is less than 25 percent, if you suffer from moderate to severe congestive heart failure, if you are not taking a beta-blocker medication, or if you did not have coronary artery bypass graft surgery when the device was implanted.[21]

WHAT HAPPENS WHEN AN ICD DISCHARGES
(DELIVERS A SHOCK)

My patients also ask:

- If I get shocked, will it hurt?
- If I get shocked in public, will I be embarrassed?
- If I get shocked, does it mean that my condition is getting worse?

As you've already read, an ICD is programmed to deliver several different levels of shocks—some intense, some moderate, some mild. Many patients say they feel dizzy or light-headed or notice rapid heartbeats just before the device discharges; others receive no warning. You may lose consciousness for a moment, but most people around you will either not notice or will think that you've fainted, which is exactly what will have happened. (For information about driving with an ICD, see p. 235). When a discharge occurs, patients report feeling anything from no pain at all to a thump on the chest to the sensation of an electrical shock. My patients have described the experience of an ICD shock in varying ways:

- "It felt something like grabbing an electrified fence."
- "It surprised me, but it didn't hurt that much."
- "It was like getting kicked in the chest—it knocked me down."
- "It didn't really hurt, but it did burn for a while."

My favorite story comes from one of my all-time favorite patients, John: "I was playing golf with my buddies, and as I hit the ball from the sixteenth tee my ICD fired. I didn't really feel much, but I blacked out for just a moment. I woke up on the ground with my friends standing over me, looking all concerned.

"I was fine. The problem was, my friends wouldn't let me retake the shot. They said, 'You did hit the ball, and you're still alive. The shot counts.' "

Not everyone bounces back as quickly as John. Some patients complain that shocks leave them feeling nervous, dizzy, weak, nauseated, or vomiting, and with a sore or tender chest. Most are awake and in the midst of an activity when they are shocked. The majority become afraid that the activity might trigger another shock, so they avoid the activity. While this may relieve anxiety in some cases, in others it promotes the development of phobias. A recent story in *The New York Times* described a seventy-one-year-old New Jersey professional woman who was so distressed by a shock she received in the shower that she couldn't step back into the stall for months (she took baths instead).[22]

I can summarize what I've learned from my patients in a few words: being shocked is usually more scary than painful. Most people are startled by the sensation, but the feeling passes quickly and within minutes you'll feel fine. Some people momentarily lose consciousness when the device discharges but awaken as soon as their heart rhythms are restored. Few describe the shock as extremely painful, but no one minimizes its impact.

Feeling nervous, fearful, or anxious after a shock is perfectly normal. After a shock, it isn't uncommon for some family members to experience higher anxiety levels than the patient.[23] As for embarrassment, reassure yourself that an ICD shock is not a spectacular event. Once your heart rhythm is restored, you'll return to normal.

ICD STORMS

When you receive a shock, it does not necessarily mean your heart condition is getting worse; it *does* mean that the ICD is doing its job. Receiving a shock does not indicate a medical emergency unless you get several in a row. That's when things get difficult.

Between 10 and 30 percent of patients experience a phenomenon called an ICD storm or electrical storm, which is when the device fires more than twice in a single twenty-four-hour period. When this happens, patients often have to check into the hospital to receive monitoring and medications that restore their normal heart rhythms.

Unlike a standard shock, an ICD storm can be terrifying. When shocks occur repeatedly and unpredictably, it's hard to tell when the flurry has ended. It's natural to fear you may be dying or that the ICD has run amok in your chest. Afterward, some patients struggle with fear, anxiety, depression, and also start to manifest symptoms of posttraumatic stress disorder (see Chapter 2). Some patients begin to engage in superstitious behaviors after a flurry of shocks: they become obsessed with the notion that if they avoid activities associated with the storm, they can avert another one. Unfortunately, it is highly unlikely that the storm was due to anything you did, or that anything you refrain from doing will fend off another one. If you become obsessed with trying to control the ICD by examining your every impulse and micromanaging every moment, you could intensify your anxiety until you're having full-blown panic attacks.

Trying to figure out why and when shocks occur will mire you in helplessness and inaction. Your energies would be better spent sitting down with your family and creating a response plan for if and when you have another storm. Here are some issues you should discuss:

KNOW WHEN TO CALL FOR HELP

If you live with and care about an ICD patient, you should be familiar with signs of trouble and know how to respond. It's wise to call the physician within twenty-four hours of a shock if the patient:

• Has received more than one shock in a day

or

• Remains unresponsive after receiving a shock

or

• Experiences continuing dizziness, lightheadedness, or fluttering in the chest after a shock

Do not leave up to the patient medical decisions such as whether or not to call the doctor: the patient is not likely to be thinking clearly after receiving a shock, and especially after an ICD storm.

- How will family members know if they should call the doctor or paramedics (see box on p. 230)?
- Who will accompany you to the doctor's office or hospital?
- On whom may you call to help loved ones left at home? If you have children, who will be able to come, in the middle of the night if necessary, and tend them until the crisis passes?
- Who will contact loved ones with updates about your condition?

BEWARE THE SICKNESS SCOREBOARD

In our work with ICD patients, Dr. Sears and I have noticed that many patients track their condition by keeping a running tally of their shocks. We call this the sickness scoreboard approach,[24] and we caution you against it because it is:

1. Fruitless and inaccurate for gauging your medical condition, and

2. Hazardous to your adjustment

Your ICD *will* sometimes deliver an inappropriate shock, so you cannot regard every shock as indicative of a dangerously abnormal heart rhythm. Shocks are sometimes caused by fractures in the wire leads and other hardware glitches that have nothing to do with the condition of your heart.

On the other hand, an absence of shocks does not mean your condition is improving. The kinds of cardiac electrical problems and rhythm disturbances that call for an ICD are usually deemed irreversible, at least at this time. Any day without a shock is a good day, but never having a shock does not mean you've been cured.

So try not to drive yourself to distraction by overinterpreting your ICD's activity. It might help to note any physical symptoms that precede a shock, such as light-headedness, dizziness, palpitations, blurred vision, fainting, or a decrease in overall physical activity. Becoming aware of these precursors can help alert you to an impending shock.

But remember that, for the most part, you are not in charge of your arrhythmia; you cannot control it. The way you choose to perceive the ICD and the role it plays in your survival will have a powerful effect on how you adjust to your illness. Make a deliberate choice to see living with an ICD as a beginning, not an ending. Put your energy into accepting that the ICD is there, standing guard over your heart. Don't squander your strength trying to interpret the device's doings—leave that to your medical team.

"ARE YOU SAYING THERE'S NOTHING I CAN DO TO AVOID GETTING SHOCKED?"

Before I answer that question, here's one for you: Which of the following situations do you think you should avoid because of having an ICD?

- Confrontations and arguments
- Being in a crowd
- Becoming overheated
- Remaining on your feet for more than three hours
- Worrying
- Having sex
- Exercising
- Job-related stress
- Gardening
- Emotional extremes, whether happy or sad
- Traveling

Answer: None of the above. No convincing proof exists that any of these activities is dangerous for ICD patients. You should, however, avoid electromagnetic fields that may interfere with your device and refrain from activities your doctor discourages. Nonetheless, you can have as fulfilling a life with the ICD as you did without it—and usually a better one. Don't make the ICD into a symbol of your illness; instead, regard it as the emblem of your deliverance. There is no magic formula of do's and don'ts to protect yourself from shocks. You have a condition that may require you to endure periodic shocks to correct your heart rhythm. The ICD is your internal SWAT team, your guardian angel, your gift of time.

At the same time, it is crucial that you manage your risk factors for heart disease. Because ischemia (when the heart needs more oxygenated blood than clogged arteries can deliver) and heart failure can alter heart rhythm patterns, ICD patients *must* be vigilant about managing their hypertension, emotions, cholesterol levels, and other risk factors that affect blood flow to the heart.

And, while you can't insure that you'll never get a shock, **taking your medications as prescribed is probably the single most effective way to decrease the odds that you'll need one.** For example, patients who take beta-blockers after their ICDs are implanted receive fewer shocks during the first year.[25] Many patients also require antiarrhythmic medications such as amiodarone. Unfortunately, some patients think the side effects from these drugs are the worst part of having an ICD. Side effects may include nausea, vomiting, headaches, weight loss, skin changes, respiratory and liver complications, depression, fatigue, and weakness.

There are emotional side effects as well. It's not unusual for patients to feel insulted, as if the necessity of taking medication is somehow an assault on their bodily integrity. I began this chapter with a quote from Deborah Daw Heffernan, whose memoir, *An Arrow Through the Heart*, is an exquisitely nuanced account of her journey to recovery from a catastrophic heart attack. In this passage, she reveals her complex relationship with the medications she must take to stay alive:

> Juliana bought me a flat plastic box with twenty-eight compartments labeled "SUN MON TUE WED THU FRI SAT" across the top and "MORN NOON EVE BED" down the side. Into these compartments we organized my medication for each week, nine pills a day. The level of detail was overwhelming; the pills were pink, white, apricot, and yellow, round, square, oval, and hexagonal. We had to squint to see the differences. Using our fingernails, we split some of the pills in half to get the right dosage, following the instructions in my discharge booklet. I sleep-walked throughout the whole sorting exercise, fighting to concentrate. My struggle was emotional; I simply could not believe that I had to live every day with this many drugs. My jaw clenched in resentment every time I snapped open one of the box's little compartments and shook the pills into my hand. . . . I could not tolerate the idea of even one more pill.[26]

If you are experiencing this real yet irrational sense of being offended by acquiescing in your own rescue, be comforted: you are not alone.

SOME TIPS FOR WHEN YOU RETURN HOME

It used to be that you could spend a week recovering in the hospital after even minor surgery, but now they send you home so quickly that it's no wonder many patients leave the hospital uncertain of what they must do to live safely with an ICD. While advice varies from doctor to doctor, here are a few universals[27]:

- For one month, refrain from lifting objects heavier than ten pounds that would require muscular exertion on the implant side. This protects you from accidentally tearing out the heart leads. Give yourself time to heal.

- For one month, do not engage in activities that require long periods of over-the-head work with the arm on the implant side (for example, painting a ceiling). Again, this will prevent you from disturbing the leads.

- Be sure to use the affected arm during normal activities to prevent your shoulder from stiffening.

- Rest assured that sleeping on the implant site is not harmful but may be uncomfortable until the wound heals.

- Avoid situations that could be dangerous were you to lose consciousness. Swimming, boating, or hiking alone is not advised. (I'll get to driving later in this chapter.)

- You may resume moderate activities, including sex, as long as they don't make you short of breath or dizzy or give you discomfort in the chest.

- Be aware that electromagnetic interference (EMI) can prevent the ICD from working properly or cause an inappropriate shock. In general, it is safe to operate household appliances that are properly grounded. However, you should avoid repairing electrical or gas-powered appliances or tools by yourself, and you should not touch a spark plug or the distributor of a running engine. Here are some common sources of electromagnetic interference:

  - Arc and resistance welding equipment

  - Induction furnaces

  - Large generators and power plants

  - Large magnets, including those used in some loudspeakers

  - Citizens band radio antennas

Also, be aware that digital cellular phones must be kept at least six inches from the implant site (this means don't carry one in your shirt pocket if it's turned on—get a belt holster instead). When using a cell phone, it's safest to use it on the ear opposite the implant site. (These warnings pertain only to digital and not to analog phones.) In addition, car-phone antennas should be mounted at least twelve inches away from where you sit.

Unlike a pacemaker, an ICD *is* likely to set off alarms when you pass through security checkpoints at airports and stores. Walking through these security systems is generally safe, but you should not lean on the antitheft mechanism or stop in the middle of its field. Also, be sure to ask airline personnel not to use a handheld screening wand to check you, as it might interfere with the ICD's ability to function. This is particularly relevant now, when airport security agents are conducting random searches of absolutely everyone—eighty-two-year-old women included. Request a manual search instead.

Finally, there's nothing dangerous about diagnostic procedures such as computerized axial tomography (CAT) scans or mammograms. But if for some reason you need an MRI—magnetic resonance imaging—and the doctor suggesting it is not aware of your heart condition, speak up! MRIs are not permitted for people who have ICDs.[28]

Even if you are exposed to a source of EMI, the ICD will usually function normally once you move away from it. But if you're in doubt about a potential source of EMI, call your nurse or physician and ask.

WHAT ABOUT DRIVING?

"Will I still be allowed to drive?"

For obvious reasons, ICD patients have unique driving concerns. Fear that an ICD might fire and cause an accident haunt both patients and family members, and lack of clarity about the issue can make relationships tense.

There are no hard-and-fast guidelines for driving with an ICD. Whether it's safe for you to drive is something you must discuss with your physicians. Everyone is different, and the decision must be made on a patient-by-patient basis. Here are some things you should think about:

- **Be honest with yourself and with your physicians.** Most physicians recommend that patients with a history of fainting, ventricular tachycardia, or ventricular fibrillation abstain from driving until it is determined that it is safe for them to do so. Typically, this means you don't get behind the wheel for the first six months after the ICD is implanted; then, your doctor reevaluates your condition. Driving is strictly prohibited until control is established over arrhythmias that can blur your vision, or cause you to become weak, light-headed, or to lose consciousness.

  Even so, research suggests that most patients resume driving before their doctors say it's safe.[29] *Don't be one of them!* Do not interpret your physician's silence on this issue as permission to drive. Be active, not passive; bring up the topic yourself. If driving is important to you—if you need to drive to get to work, or perform your job, or buy groceries, or care for your elderly parents, tell your physician. Then wait until he or she gives you the go-ahead before getting back behind the wheel. Your own safety and that of your loved ones is riding on it.

- **Know the facts.** In cases where a driver is suddenly incapacitated due to medical reasons, less than 2 percent result in death or injury to other drivers or bystanders (innocent or not).[30] Researchers have concluded that when a driver's ICD fires and causes him or her to have an accident, the odds against harming someone else are about 45,000 to one.[31] These are actually great odds, especially when you consider your chances of dying as a result of a gun accident (2,500 to one), passenger aircraft crash (20,000 to one), or an asteroid or comet crashing to earth (20,000 to one).[32]

- **Use common sense.** A few commonsense precautions are worth taking whenever you get behind the wheel:

  - Limit your driving to local streets.

  - Avoid driving on highways.

  - Stay in the right lane so you can exit easily if you need to.

  - Don't take trips that require you to drive for hours at a time.

- **Recognize that this is a family decision.** Include family members in the discussion of whether you should resume driving, and when. Although some of them may be overprotective, don't ignore their feelings. Your illness is stressful for them, and their concern for your safety (and theirs if they're passengers in a car you're driving) should be taken seriously.

WHAT ABOUT SEX?

None of my patients has ever reported that his or her ICD fired during sex, but that doesn't prevent them from worrying. This is how Dave put it: "I used to worry I might have a heart attack during sex and it would traumatize my wife. Now that I have this gizmo, I worry that I might electrocute her!"

Fortunately for Dave and his wife, this fear is unfounded. I can't back this up with statistics because we don't have definitive data on the incidence of ICD firings during sex. But I can say that I've never heard of a partner being harmed by an ICD discharge during sex—not from my patients, nor from others—so I am deducing that this simply doesn't happen. More important, I can offer this reassurance: if your ICD fires and you're touching someone, the risk to that person is minuscule. The most he or she might feel is a tiny static electricity kind of pop—a bit surprising, perhaps, but certainly not painful.

Of course, your sexual adjustment after receiving an ICD encompasses more than concerns about shocks. Everything covered in Chapter 9 applies here, too. Remember also that the fact that you were eligible for an ICD means you've probably had an extended struggle with heart disease. If so, the severity of your illness and the medications you take to control it probably drain you of sexual energy. Your interest in sex may also diminish if you're self-conscious about the small bulge in the implant area.

WHAT ABOUT PREGNANCY AND CHILDBIRTH?

Younger women who have received ICDs often worry about whether or not pregnancy and childbirth are safe, both for themselves and the baby. Dr. Samuel F. Sears and associates (including my daughter Rebecca, a doctoral candidate in clinical psychology) reviewed the medical literature on this topic and concluded that there is little risk to mother or child as a result of ICD implantation, discharges, or potential malfunction.[33] The main pregnancy issue involves blood flow to the fetus. When an ICD delivers a shock to a pregnant woman, it temporarily lowers her blood pressure after the shock, and the question is whether this will reduce blood flow to the placenta and the fetus. So far, the prognosis is good: when a woman does receive an ICD shock during labor or delivery, no complications occur either in mother or child. And, contrary to what your intuition might tell you, neither pregnancy nor delivery increases the odds that an ICD will discharge.

CONNECT WITH OTHER ICD PATIENTS

Don't retreat into a shell-shocked cocoon: reach out and talk with people who have learned to live with an ICD. Your physician will know about support groups in your area, as do the major manufacturers of the device—Medtronic, St. Jude Medical, and Guidant—whose headquarters and Web sites provide help and support group information as well (see Resources).

If you are like the vast majority of ICD patients, you'll be tending your heart for the rest of your life. You may be in for return trips to the hospital, new (and improved) medications and devices, and occasional surgery to replace your ICD's generator and adjust its lead system.

Receiving—and accepting—an ICD is one more step in your journey. It is neither a calamity nor a cure: it cannot prevent your heart from beating erratically, but it *will* correct arrhythmias when they occur. It is a great and bountiful gift, the gift of life itself. As with any gift, the wisest response is to accept it wholeheartedly and gratefully.

AFTERWORD

Writing the final words of this book is like relishing the last morsel of a favorite meal; I am filled with contentment to have helped readers by sharing the wisdom of exceptional heart patients.

Yet even in this moment of satisfaction, I see that there will always be more for me to learn and teach. As this edition goes to press, new developments offer hope for thriving with heart disease. Off-pump coronary bypass surgery, in which a surgeon performs the procedure on a beating heart, eliminates the need to place the patient on a ventilator and may reduce the cognitive decline associated with spending time on a heart-lung machine. Research is homing in on the kinds of inflammation that may be the main culprits in coronary heart disease. Statins, a class of drugs known for lowering cholesterol, are suddenly doing a lot more than that—scientists think they may also treat and perhaps even prevent diseases such as multiple sclerosis, cancer, and Alzheimer's. And, with the expanding use of left-ventricular assist devices, some patients who might have needed transplants—or died waiting for them—now have a chance to hold on to their hearts as well as their lives. Every day brings an encouraging breakthrough, an unexpected benefit, an invigorating jolt of hope.

I rejoice that there seems to be no end to the stream of new treatments to help heart patients thrive. The coming decade will see the largest, most diverse population of heart patients ever, and learning from them and their families is the zenith of my professional fulfillment. I hope this book has been helpful to you, and welcome your comments, questions, and responses. I want to know your experiences, what you and your loved ones are learning on your journey of living with heart disease.

Please contact me:

- Through my Web site: www.ThrivingWithHeartDisease.com
- By e-mail: wsotile@attglobal.net
- Or by writing to me:

Wayne M. Sotile, Ph.D.

Sotile Psychological Associates

1396 Old Mill Circle

Winston-Salem, NC 27103

I am a better person because of the exceptional heart patients who have graced me with their candor, constancy, and valor; it is my privilege to keep their counsel. In facing death, they have taught me how to live, and the most galvanizing lesson I've learned is that we should stop biding our time and spend more of it rejoicing.

APPENDIX

MEDICATIONS

The charts that follow list medications commonly used to treat heart disease. Chart I lists medications prescribed to treat depression; Chart II, antianxiety medications; and Chart III, cardiovascular medications. The charts integrate information from a variety of sources which you may consult for more details about each medicine's uses, dosage range, side effects, and interactions with other medicines.[1] The list is a long one but is unavoidably incomplete, as new medications hit the market every day.

Read the charts and circle any medications you are taking. You'll see there are numerous side effects noted in the Comments columns. Don't panic when you read these—drug manufacturers are required to list any and all side effects that could possibly occur, no matter how rare or innocuous they may be. Many are seldom if ever experienced by most of a medication's users.

Of course, the information in these charts is for educational purposes only and **not meant to substitute for a consultation with your physician.** Also, please note that a medication's side effects vary from patient to patient and that many side effects are possible in addition to those that are listed. If you develop bothersome reactions to a drug, contact your physician: only he or she can make informed decisions about your medications.

The more medications you take and the higher the dosages, the more likely you are to experience unwanted side effects. Even if this happens, **do not stop taking your medicines**—talk with your physician instead. The great news is that, as you can see, many drugs are available to treat just about any medical problem. If you are concerned about any aspect of your medication regimen, again—speak with your doctor.

CHART I: ANTIDEPRESSANTS

Selective Serotonin Reuptake Inhibitors (SSRIs)

BRAND NAME	GENERIC NAME	COMMENTS
Celexa . . . . .citalopram		Few cardiovascular complications, but long-term effects on myocardium (middle layer of heart muscle) as yet undetermined. If your physician prescribes an SSRI, be sure he or she knows you have heart disease. May cause nausea, skin rash, diarrhea, anxiety, headaches, tremor, constipation, dry mouth, drowsiness, or sexual dysfunction, including diminised sex drive and disturbed orgasm and/or ejaculation. Recent research shows **sertraline (Zoloft)** to be safe for use soon after MI or unstable angina.[2]
Lexapro . . . . .escitalopram		
Luvox . . . . .fluvoxamine		
Paxil . . . . .paroxetine		
Prozac . . . . .fluoxetine		
Zoloft . . . . .sertraline		

Serotonin and Norepinephrine Reuptake Inhibitors (SNRIs)

BRAND NAME	GENERIC NAME	COMMENTS
Desyrel . . . . .trazodone		May cause weakness, dry mouth, dizziness, constipation, anxiety, insomnia, drowsiness, and sexual dysfunction. Fewer sexual side effects with **nefazodone (Serzone),** but may cause unwanted drop in blood pressure and so is prescribed for heart patients cautiously. **Trazodone (Desyrel)** may cause painful, prolonged erections (priapism). **Venlafaxine (Effexor, Effexor XR)** may elevate heart rate and blood pressure, especially at high doses; discontinuing it abruptly may cause temporary physical symptoms.
Effexor . . . . .venlafaxine		
Effexor XR . . . . . . .venlafaxine, sustained-release		
Serzone . . . . .nefazodone hydrochloride		

Dopamine Reuptake Inhibitors

BRAND NAME	GENERIC NAME	COMMENTS
Wellbutrin	bupropion	May cause insomnia, restlessness, headache, constipation, loss of appetite, tremor, dry mouth, increased sweating, nausea, or vomiting. Low levels of sexual side effects, with some evidence that these drugs may enhance sexual performance. Very few cardiovascular problems, but tell your physician you're a heart patient before taking any of these medicines. The only significant side effect is the possibility of inducing seizures at high dosages or if consumed with alcohol.
Wellbutrin SR	bupropion, sustained-release	

Tricyclics

BRAND NAME	GENERIC NAME	COMMENTS
Anafranil	clomipramine	Many cardiovascular complications, including hypotension, tachycardia, and conduction block; also dizziness, sedation, blurred vision, dry mouth, constipation, urinary retention, and sexual dysfunction. Increases skin sensitivity to sunlight. If your physician suggests you take one of these medications, be sure to inform him or her that you are a heart patient.
Asendin	amoxapine	
Aventyl	nortriptyline	
Elavil	amitriptyline	
Endep	amitriptyline	
Etrafon	amitriptyline + perphenazine	
Etrafon-A	amitriptyline + perphenazine	
Etrafon-Forte	amitriptyline + perphenazine	
Limbitrol	amitriptyline + chlordiazepoxide	
Norpramin	desipramine	
Pamelor	nortriptyline	
Sinequan	doxepin	
Surmontil	trimipramine	
Tofranil	imipramine	
Vivactil	protriptyline	

CHART II: ANTIANXIETY MEDICATIONS

Selective Serotonin Reuptake Inhibitors (SSRIs)

BRAND NAME	GENERIC NAME	COMMENTS
Celexa ....citalopram		In addition to treating depression, these medications are effective against anxiety, obsessive-compulsive disorder, and post-traumatic stress disorder. For side effects and cardiovascular risks, see "SSRIs," p. 242.
Lexapro ....escitalopram		
Luvox ....fluvoxamine		
Paxil ....paroxetine		
Prozac ....fluoxetine		
Zoloft ....sertraline		

Serotonin and Norepinephrine Reuptake Inhibitors (SNRIs)

BRAND NAME	GENERIC NAME	COMMENTS
Desyrel ....trazodone		In addition to treating depression, used variously to treat anxiety disorders and insomnia, alone or with an SSRI. For side effects and cardiovascular risks, see "SNRIs," p. 242.
Effexor ....venlafaxine		
Effexor XR ....venlafaxine, sustained-release		
Serzone ....nefazodone hydrochloride		

Azaspirone

BRAND NAME	GENERIC NAME	COMMENTS
BuSpar ....buspirone		Does not cause drowsiness; is nonaddictive. No particular cardiovascular risks. May cause dizziness, nausea, light-headedness.

Tricyclics

BRAND NAME	GENERIC NAME	COMMENTS
Anafranil . . . . .clomipramine		Used variously to treat obsessive-compulsive disorder, panic disorder, generalized anxiety disorder, and phobias. For side effects and cardiovascular risks, see "Tricyclics," page 243.
Aventyl . . . . .nortriptyline		
Norpramin . . . . . . .desipramine		
Pamelor . . . . .nortriptyline		
Tofranil . . . . .imipramine		
Vivactil . . . . .protriptyline		

Benzodiazepines

BRAND NAME	GENERIC NAME	COMMENTS
Ativan . . . . .lorazepam		Side effects may include hypotension (low blood pressure), nausea, dizziness, and nervousness. Chronic use may lead to addiction.
Dalmane . . . . .flurazepam		
Doral . . . . .quazepam		
Gen-Xene . . . . .clorazepate		
Halcion . . . . .triazolam		
Klonopin . . . . .clonazepam		
Librium . . . . .chlordiazepoxide		
Paxipam . . . . .halazepam		
ProSom . . . . .estazolam		
Restoril . . . . .temazepam		
Serax . . . . .oxazepam		
Tranxene . . . . .clorazepate		
Tranxene-SD . . . . . .clorazepate		
Valium . . . . .diazepam		
Xanax . . . . .alprazolam		

CHART III: CARDIOVASCULAR MEDICATIONS

Diuretics

Commonly known as water pills, these medicines increase urine flow and help eliminate excess fluid. Some cause vasodilation (expansion of blood vessels). Decreased body fluid and dilated blood vessels reduce blood pressure; still, diuretics are more commonly used to treat heart failure than hypertension.

Diuretics

BRAND NAME	GENERIC NAME	COMMENTS
Aldactazide	spironolactone + hydrochlorothiazide	May cause either retention or loss of potassium, lower blood pressure, and deplete body fluids. May increase uric acid levels, resulting in gout. May affect sex drive and sexual performance. If you take a diuretic, be sure to check your potassium levels regularly. High blood levels of potassium may cause weakness, drowsiness, and muscle pain or cramping.
Aldactone	spironolactone	
Bumex	bumetanide	
Demadex	torsemide	
Diuril	chlorothiazine	
Dyazide	hydrochlorothiazide + triamterene	
Dyrenium	triamterene	
Edecrin	ethacrynic acid	
Esidrix	hydrochlorothiazide	
HydroDIURIL	hydrochlorothiazide	
Hygroton	chlorthalidone	
Lasix	furosemide	
Lozol	indapamide	
Maxzide	hydrochlorothiazide + triamterene	
Maxzide-25 MG	hydrochlorothiazide + triamterene	
Midmar	amiloride	
Moduretic	amiloride + hydrochlorothiazide	
Mykrox	metolazone	
Thalitone	chlorthalidone	
Zaroxolyn	metolazone	

Beta-Blockers

These mitigate the effects of adrenaline, thereby strengthening cardiac contractions and lowering heart rate and blood pressure. Taking a beta-blocker during or immediately after a heart attack may reduce heart muscle damage. Taking a beta-blocker also reduces your risk of having a repeat cardiac event. New studies show beta-blockers to be effective in treating atrial fibrillation.[3] Beta-blockers are sometimes used to reduce anxiety.

Beta-Blockers

BRAND NAME	GENERIC NAME	COMMENTS
Betapace	sotalol	Because beta-blockers reduce the amount of blood the heart pumps with each beat, patients with severe heart failure or very slow heart rates should use these medicines with caution. Consult your physician when discontinuing this or any medication. When you stop beta-blocker treatment, reduce the dosage gradually over one to two weeks. Most common side effects include impotence, loss of sex drive, fatigue, nightmares, insomnia and other sleep problems, and difficulties with concentration and mental alertness at higher doses. Some side effects mimic symptoms of depression, which affects between 4 percent and 12 percent of users. Less common side effects include hypotension (low blood pressure), slowed heart rate, dizziness or fainting, and cold hands, feet, ears, or nose.
Betapace AF	sotalol	
Blocadren	timolol	
Coreg	carvedilol	
Corgard	nadolol	
Corzide	nadolol + bendroflumethiazide	
Inderal	propranolol	
Inderide	propranolol hydrochloride + hydrochlorothiazide	
Lopressor	metoprolol	
Normodyne	labetalol	
Sectral	acebutolol	
Sorine	sotalol	
Tenoretic	atenolol + chlorthalidone	
Tenormin	atenolol	
Toprol-XL	metoprolol	
Trandate	labetalol	
Visken	pindolol	
Zebeta	bisoprolol	

Calcium Channel Blockers

These limit the cardiac and vascular smooth muscles' absorption of calcium. These medicines expand both coronary and peripheral arteries, reduce squeezing of cardiac muscle, lower blood pressure, and reduce erratic heart rhythms. They are prescribed to treat angina and high blood pressure, and to prevent patients from suffering repeat heart attacks. New studies show calcium channel blockers to be effective in treating atrial fibrillation.[4]

Calcium Channel Blockers

BRAND NAME	GENERIC NAME	COMMENTS
Adalat	nifedipine	Mild medications with few bothersome side effects, especially at lower dosages and with younger patients. At higher dosages, side effects may include dizziness or light-headedness; fluid retention in legs, feet, or hands; weakness or fatigue; facial flushing; tachycardia; palpitations; headache; low blood pressure; dizziness; and fainting. In patients with ventricular problems, may cause heart failure or heart block (conduction mishap that results in delay or inability of an electrical impulse to reach the ventricles). In some cases, may cause anxiety or depression.
Adalat CC	nifedipine	
Calan	verapamil	
Cardene	nicardipine	
Cardene SR	nicardipine	
Cardizem	diltiazem	
Cardizem CD	diltiazem	
Cardizem SR	diltiazem	
Cartia-XT	diltiazem	
Dilacor	diltiazem	
Dilacor XR	diltiazem	
Diltia XT	diltiazem	
DynaCirc	isradipine	
Isoptin	verapamil	
Lotrel	amlodipine + benazepril hydrochloride	
Norvasc	amlodipine	
Plendil	felodipine	
Procardia	nifedipine	
Procardia XL	nifedipine	
Sular	nisoldipine	
Tiamate	diltiazem	
Tiazac	diltiazem	
Verelan	verapamil	

Alpha-Blockers
These reduce blood pressure by widening blood vessels, and sometimes also improve urinary flow.

Alpha-Blockers

BRAND NAME	GENERIC NAME	COMMENTS
Aldomet	methyldopa	Side effects may include headaches, weakness, dizziness, fainting, and dry mouth, especially with the first few doses. In some cases, may cause anxiety or depression.
Cardura	doxazosin	
Catapres	clonidine	
Hytrin	terazosin	
Minipress	prazosin	

Angiotensin II Blockers
These lower blood pressure by blocking the effects of blood-vessel-constricting hormones. They are frequently used to treat heart failure.

Angiotensin II Blockers

BRAND NAME	GENERIC NAME	COMMENTS
Atacand	candesartan	Angiotensin II blockers do not cause coughing, as ACE inhibitors do. Some studies suggest that **telmisartan, losartan, irbesartan,** and **candesartan** are less effective in African Americans. Side effects may include respiratory infection, changes in urinary frequency, dizziness, and gastrointestinal (GI) upset. If you are taking an angiotensin II blocker and exercise strenuously in hot weather, the drug may cause your blood pressure to drop rapidly. In some cases, it may cause anxiety or depression.
Avalide	irbesartan hydrochlorothiazide	
Avapro	irbesartan	
Benicar	olmesartan	
Cozaar	losartan potassium	
Diovan	valsartan	
Diovan HCT	valsartan hydrochlorothiazide	
Hyzaar	losartan potassium + hydrochlorothiazide	
Micardis	telmisartan	
Teveten	eprosartan mesylate	

Blood Thinners (Anticoagulants and Antiplatelet Agents)
These either prevent platelets from forming a clot (aspirin) or interfere with blood's normal coagulation (all others). These medicines are taken by persons whose heart valves have been replaced with mechanical ones, and by those who suffer atrial fibrillation to ward off stroke, cardiomyopathy, and poor ventricular function. Also used to treat some patients with coronary artery stents or recent clots in coronary arteries.

Blood Thinners (Anticoagulants)

BRAND NAME	GENERIC NAME	COMMENTS
Adprin-B . . . . .aspirin		These medicines slow blood clotting, so be sure your dentist and all your physicians know you're taking them. Also be careful when shaving and in situations where you might cut yourself. Must be taken exactly as prescribed.
Arthritis Pain Formula . . . . .aspirin		
Ascriptin . . . . .aspirin		
Aspergum . . . . . . .aspirin		
Asprimox . . . . .aspirin		**Warfarin, anisindione,** and **dicumarol** interfere with absorption of vitamin K, which affects clotting. If you take these medicines, your blood must be tested periodically to monitor its clotting factor (prothrombin time). You should stay away from green, leafy vegetables such as spinach and kale; avoid alcohol and physically jarring activities such as horseback riding. Side effects may include bruising or unusual bleeding, rash, diarrhea, nausea, or upset stomach.
Bayer . . . . .aspirin		
Bufferin . . . . .aspirin		
Coumadin . . . . .warfarin		
dicumarol (generic only) . . . . .dicumarol		
Easprin . . . . .aspirin		
Ecotrin . . . . .aspirin		
Empirin . . . . .aspirin		**Heparin,** administered by injection, acts swiftly.
Genprin . . . . .aspirin		
Heartline . . . . .aspirin		
heparin (generic only) . . . . .heparin		
Magnaprin . . . . . . .aspirin		
Miradon . . . . .anisindione		
Norwich . . . . .aspirin		
Plavix . . . . .clopidogrel bisulfate		
St. Joseph . . . . .aspirin		
Ticlid . . . . .ticlopidine		
Trental . . . . .pentoxifylline		

Rhythm Stabilizers

These treat severe arrhythmias by either reducing sensitivity of heart tissue to nerve pulses or slowing the rate at which pulses move through the tissue.

Rhythm Stabilizers

BRAND NAME	GENERIC NAME
Cardioquin	quinidine
Cordarone	amiodarone
Lanoxin	digoxin
Mexitil	mexiletine
Norpace	disopyramide
Norpace CR	disopyramide
Pacerone	amiodarone
Procan	procainamide
Procan-SR	procainamide
Pronestyl	procainamide
Pronestyl-SR	procainamide
Quinaglute Dura-Tabs	quinidine
Quinalan	quinidine
Quinidex Extentabs	quinidine
Quinora	quinidine
Rythmol	propafenone
Sectral	acebutolol
Tambocor	flecainide

COMMENTS

A large percentage of persons taking rhythm stabilizers suffer side effects, some of them onerous. May include fatigue, unusual involuntary movements or tics, weakness, reduced sex drive, sleep disturbance, GI upset, and dry eyes.

Amiodarone: In some cases, leads to lung damage, impaired thyroid function, slowed heart rate, arrhythmia, heart block, liver damage, vision problems, and sun sensitivity.

Disopyramide: May cause anxiety, chills, drowsiness, GI upset, weakness, and urinary difficulty. May also worsen heart failure or trigger dangerously low blood pressure.

Procainamide: Common side effects include appetite loss, GI upset, joint and muscle pain. In some cases, may affect bone marrow and reduce white blood cell count.

Quinidine: May cause GI upset and oral problems, including dry mouth and periodontal disease. See your dentist regularly when taking quinidine. High dosages may lead to hearing loss, ringing in ears, and vision problems.

Flecainide: May cause dizziness or disorientation, making it difficult to drive or perform other complex tasks.

Cholesterol-Lowering Medications
These work in various ways to reduce LDL (bad) cholesterol and triglyceride levels, and/or increase HDL (good) cholesterol levels. They are prescribed for persons whose levels are mildly elevated as well as for those with higher numbers, and for patients with a history of heart disease, heart attack, or bypass surgery. These medications break down into three categories: **statins, bile acid sequestrates,** and **dietary supplements. Statins** work by slowing a liver enzyme that produces LDL cholesterol, which delivers fat to arteries. Statins also modestly increase production of HDL, which removes fat from arteries. **Bile acid sequestrates** work by absorbing bile acids—which contain cholesterol—in the bowel, where the medication remains. **Dietary supplements** work by lowering LDL and triglyceride levels while raising HDL levels.

Cholesterol-Lowering Medications

BRAND NAME	GENERIC NAME	COMMENTS

Statins

BRAND NAME	GENERIC NAME	COMMENTS
Advicor	lovastatin + niacin	May aggravate or cause liver disease in persons who consume large quantities of alcohol. May raise liver enzyme count, cause muscle weakness and aches, sun sensitivity, and impotence. Can cause skeletal muscle damage. May cause GI upset, sleep disturbance, or depression. Common side effects associated with specific brands include headache **(Lipitor)**; respiratory infection **(Lescol, Lescol XL)**; stomach pain, cramps, gas, and constipation **(Mevacor)**; flushing **(Advicor)**. Persons taking statins must have their blood checked regularly.
Lescol	fluvastatin	
Lescol XL	fluvastatin	
Lipitor	atorvastatin	
Lopid	gemfibrozil	
Mevacor	lovastatin	
Pravachol	pravastatin	
Zocor	simvastatin	
Crestor	Promising new statin, due out in 2003; early research suggests superior ability to lower lipids.	

Bile Acid Sequestrates

Colestid . . . . .colestipol hydrochloride

LoCHOLEST
Light . . . . .cholestyramine

LoCHOLEST
Prevalite . . . . .cholestyramine

Prevalite . . . . .cholestyramine

Questran . . . . .cholestyramine

Questran Light . . . .cholestyramine

WelChol . . . . .colesevelam

Many GI difficulties, including nausea, abdominal pain, indigestion, and constipation. May cause impotence.

Dietary Supplements

Cholestin . . . .(various)

Niacin (nicotinic acid) . . . .(various)

Cholestin's long-term safety has not been tested.

Niacin's side effects may include flushing and elevation of liver enzyme levels and blood sugar. Extremely high doses may cause liver damage, peptic ulcers, and blood sugar fluctuations.

Nitrates

These temporarily relieve chest pain by dilating blood vessels, enabling more oxygen to reach the heart. They also prevent platelets from adhering to artery walls. In tablet form, nitrates dissolve rapidly and take effect in thirty to ninety seconds; their effect lasts for ten to thirty minutes. Even faster-acting nitrates are available in spray form. Longer-lasting nitrates, whose effects last up to several hours, come as pills, patches, and ointments; also available as a transdermal patch.

Nitrates

BRAND NAME	GENERIC NAME	COMMENTS
Deponit	nitroglycerin	**Mixing any form of nitrate with drugs that enhance sexual functioning, such as Viagra (sildenafil), is *dangerous*.**
Imdur	isosorbide mononitrate	
ISMO	isosorbide mononitrate	
Isordil	isosorbide dinitrate	**Nitrates** may cause flushing and headache, tachycardia, palpitations, and dizziness or fainting if you take them and stand up quickly. No psychiatric side effects.
Minitran	nitroglycerin	
Monoket	isosorbide mononitrate	
Nitrek	nitroglycerin	
Nitro Tab	nitroglycerin	
Nitro-Bid	nitroglycerin	
Nitro-Derm	nitroglycerin	
Nitrodisc	nitroglycerin	
Nitro-Dur	nitroglycerin	
Nitrogard	nitroglycerin	
Nitroglyn	nitroglycerin	
Nitrol	nitroglycerin	
Nitrolingual	nitroglycerin	
Nitrolingual spray	nitroglycerin	
Nitrong	nitroglycerin	
NitroQuick	nitroglycerin	
Nitrostat	nitroglycerin	
Nitro-Time	nitroglycerin	
Sorbitrate	isosorbide dinitrate	
Transderm-Nitro	nitroglycerin	

Cardiac Strengtheners

These intensify heart contractions and control rhythm disturbances by decreasing ventricular rate in episodes of fibrillation, flutter, and tachycardia. They also improve circulation and are often prescribed for heart failure and rapid heartbeat.

Cardiac Strengtheners

BRAND NAME	GENERIC NAME	COMMENTS
Dobutrex	dobutamine (administered via injection)	At high dosages, may cause nausea, vomiting, tinted vision, arrhythmia, and dizziness. Pulse should be monitored daily. **Digoxin** may cause apathy and confusion.
Lanoxicaps	digoxin	
Lanoxin	digoxin	

RESOURCES

Please note that all Web site URLs are subject to change.

HEALTH AND HEART DISEASE

American College of Cardiology
Heart House
9111 Old Georgetown Road
Bethesda, MD 20814-1699
Telephone: (800) 253-4636;
(301) 897-5400
Web site: www.acc.org
Professional organization of cardio-vascular physicians and scientists.

American Heart Association
7272 Greenville Avenue
Dallas, TX 75231
Telephone: (800) 242-8721
[(800) AHA-USA1]; (214) 373-6300
Web site: www.americanheart.org

American Medical Association
515 N. State Street
Chicago, IL 60610
Telephone: (312) 464-5000
Web site: www.ama-assn.org
Professional organization of medical doctors.

Health Canada
A.L. 0900 C2
Ottawa, Ontario K1A 0K9
Canada
Telephone: (613) 957-2991
Web site: www.hc-sc.gc.ca

National Black Women's Health Project
600 Pennsylvania Avenue, S.E.
Suite 310
Washington, DC 20003
Telephone: (202) 548-4000
Web site: www.blackwomenshealth.org

National Coalition for Women with Heart Disease
818 18th Street, N.W., Suite 730
Washington, DC 20006
Telephone: (202) 728-7199
Web site: www.womenheart.org

The National Heart, Lung, and Blood Institute
Information Center
P.O. Box 30105
Bethesda, MD 20824-0105
Telephone: (800) 575-9355
[(800) 575-WELL]
Web site: www.nhlbi.nih.gov
Part of the National Institutes of Health.

National Women's Health Network
514 10th Street, N.W., Suite 400
Washington, DC 20004
Telephone: (202) 628-7814 (health information); (202) 347-1140 (administration)
Web site: www.womenshealth network.org
The only national nonprofit organization devoted to women's health, it accepts no donations from drug or tobacco companies or manufacturers of medical devices.

Texas Heart Institute
P.O. Box 20345
Houston, TX 77225-0345
Telephone: (800) 292-2221;
(832) 355-6536
Web site: www.texasheartinstitute.org

The Vascular Disease Foundation
3333 South Wadsworth Boulevard
Suite B-104-37
Lakewood, CO 80227
Telephone: (866) 723-4636;
(303) 949-8337
Web site: www.vdf.org
Nonprofit organization dedicated to providing information about vascular disease. Publishes Keeping in Circulation, *a free quarterly available both in print and online formats (see Newsletters, p. 262).*

Women's Health Initiative
6705 Rockledge Drive
Suite 300, MSC-7966, RKLI
Bethesda, MD 20892-7966
Telephone: (301) 402-2900
Web site: www.nhlbi.nih.gov/whi
Part of the National Institutes of Health.

CARDIAC REHABILITATION PROGRAMS

American Association of Cardiovascular and Pulmonary Rehabilitation
401 North Michigan Avenue
Suite 2200
Chicago, IL 60611-4267
Telephone: (312) 321-5146
Web site: www.aacvpr.org

The Wake Forest Cardiac Rehabilitation Program
Department of Medicine/Health & Exercise Science
P.O. Box 7628, Reynolda Station
Winston-Salem, NC 27109
Telephone: (336) 758-5395
Web site: www.wfu.edu/Academic-departments/Health-and-Exercise-Science/cardiac.htm

MARITAL AND FAMILY HEALTH

American Association for Marriage and Family Therapy
112 South Alfred Street
Alexandria, VA 22314-3061
Telephone: (703) 838-9808
Web site: www.aamft.org
Can refer you to a qualified family therapist in your area.

The Coalition for Marriage, Family, and Couples Education
5310 Belt Road, N.W.
Washington, DC 20015-1961
Telephone: (202) 362-3332
Web site: www.smartmarriages.com
Can refer you to seminars and courses that teach marriage and family skills.

The Association for Couples in Marriage Enrichment
P.O. Box 10596
Winston-Salem, NC 27108
Telephone: (800) 634-8325;
(336) 724-1526
Web site: www.bettermarriages.org
Good source of information on marriage enrichment and education programs.

MENTAL HEALTH

American Psychiatric Association
1400 K Street, N.W.
Washington, DC 20005
Telephone: (888) 357-7924
Web site: www.psych.org

American Psychological Association
750 First Street, N.E.
Washington, DC 20002-4242
Telephone: (800) 374-2721;
(202) 336-5510
TDD/TTY: (202) 336-6123
Web site: www.apa.org

Anxiety Disorders Association of America
8730 Georgia Avenue, Suite 600
Silver Spring, MD 20910
Telephone: (240) 485-1001
Web site: www.adaa.org

National Institute of Mental Health
Public Inquiries
6001 Executive Boulevard, Room 8184, MSC 9663
Bethesda, MD 20892-9663
Telephone: (301) 443-4513
Web site: www.nimh.nih.gov

SUPPORT GROUPS

American Self-Help Group Clearinghouse
100 E. Hanover Avenue, Suite 202
Cedar Knolls, NJ 07927-2020
Telephone: (973) 326-6789
Web site: www.selfhelpgroups.org

MEDICATION

American Society of Health-System Pharmacists
7272 Wisconsin Avenue
Bethesda, MD 20814
Telephone: (301) 657-3000
Web site: www.safemedication.com

www.rxlist.com
Owned and operated by Neil Sandow, licensed California pharmacist, this online directory of more than four thousand brand-name and generic medications allows you to search for information on a specific drug or a category of drugs.

Food and Drug Administration
5600 Fishers Lane
Rockville, MD 20857-0001
Web site: www.fda.gov

NUTRITION

American Dietetic Association
216 West Jackson Boulevard
Chicago, IL 60606-6995
Telephone: (312) 899-0040
Web site: www.eatright.org

SMOKING CESSATION

Action on Smoking and Health
2013 H Street, N.W.
Washington, DC 20006
Telephone: (202) 659-4310
Web site: www.ash.org

American Cancer Society
1599 Clifton Road, NE
Atlanta, GA 30329-4251
Telephone: (800) 227-2345
Web site: www.cancer.org

American Lung Association
61 Broadway, 6th Floor
New York, NY 10006
Telephone: (800) 586-4872;
(212) 315-8700
Web site: www.lungusa.org

IMPLANTABLE CARDIOVERTER DEFIBRILLATOR (ICD)

St. Jude Medical
Telephone: (800) 777-2237
Web site: www.sjm.com

Guidant
Telephone: (800) CARDIAC [(800) 227-3422]
Web site: www.guidant.com

Medtronic
Telephone: (800) 328-2518
Web site: www.medtronic.com

St. Jude Medical, Guidant, and **Medtronic** all manufacture ICDs and operate Web sites that provide information about living with heart illness in general and ICDs in particular. The sites are great for learning about your device, its capabilities, and what to expect as an ICD recipient.

www.implantable.com
Site is intended as a clearinghouse for information related to implantable devices and is geared primarily toward medical professionals.

OTHER WEB SITES

Please note that all Web site URLs are subject to change.

www.4hcm.org
Web site of the Hypertrophic Cardiomy-opathy Association, a nonprofit organization that provides information and support to patients and families. Or you can write to HCMA, P.O. Box 306, Hibernia, NJ 07842; or phone (973) 983-7429.

www.cachnet.org
Web site cosponsored by the Canadian Adult Congenital Heart Network and Toronto Congenital Cardiac Centre for Adults at the University of Toronto. Provides information and links to helpful Internet sources for adult patients with congenital heart defects and their care providers; also publishes an online newsletter, The Beat, *which can be accessed by visiting the site.*

www.healthy.net
General information on monitoring your own health, sponsored by Health-WorldOnline.

www.heartcenteronline.com
Solid information for loved ones of heart patients, with pointers on stress management.

www.heartdisease.about.com
Operated by Medscape, this patient-oriented site provides information on all aspects of heart illness.

www.heartdisease.com
Provides links to information about heart illness.

www.heartfailure.org
Information on heart failure.

www.heartinfo.org
Independent, educational site.

www.hrt.org
Connects you with Online Journal of Cardiology.

www.hsforum.com
Provides information on cardiac surgery, published by the International Society for Minimally Invasive Cardiac Surgery.

www.mayoclinic.com
Site of the world-famous Mayo Health Clinic in Rochester, Minnesota.

www.medem.com
Devoted to "medical empowerment" and operated by the American Medical Association in collaboration with various professional societies.

www.medscape.com
Now affiliated with WebMD; provides a wide variety of breaking medical news and information.

www.naspe.org
Web site of the North American Society of Pacing and Electrophysiology, profes-sional society of electrophysiologists. Site focuses on heart rhythm and arrhythmia information. The section devoted to patients' stories can be inspiring.

www.pulsus.com/cardiol/links.htm
Links to various cardiology journals; for links to journals in other specialties, go to www.pulsus.com.

www.ThrivingWithHeartDisease.com
My Web site, offering advice and information for heart patients and their loved ones.

www.webmd.com
General health information.

NEWSLETTERS

Caregiving
Tad Publishing Company
P.O. Box 224
Park Ridge, IL 60068
Telephone: (847) 823-0639
Web site: www.caregiving.com

The Cleveland Clinic Heart Advisor
Subscription Service
P.O. Box 420235
Palm Coast, FL 32142-0235
Telephone: (800) 829-2506

Keeping in Circulation
The Vascular Disease Foundation
3333 South Wadsworth Boulevard
Suite B-104-37
Lakewood, CO 80227
Telephone: (866) 723-4636;
(303) 949-8337
Web site: www.vdf.org

Harvard Women's Health Watch
Harvard Health Publications
10 Shattuck Street, Suite 612
Boston, MA 02115
Web site: www.health.harvard.edu/
section.cfm?id=18

**The Johns Hopkins Medical Letter,
Health After 50**
P.O. Box 420179
Palm Coast, FL 32142
Telephone: (386) 447-6313
Web site: www.hopkinsafter50.com

NOTES

Chapter 1: Begin the Journey

1. J. Denollet and D. L. Brutsaert, "Personality, Disease Severity, and the Risk of Long-Term Cardiac Events in Patients with Decreased Ejection Fraction After Myocardial Infarction," *Circulation* 97 (1998): 167–173; S. Friedman, "Cardiac Disease, Anxiety, and Sexual Functioning," *The American Journal of Cardiology* 86, no. 2A (July 20, 2000): 46F–50F; T. Rutledge, W. Linden, and R. F. Davies, "Psychological Risk Factors May Moderate Pharmacological Treatment Effects Among Ischemic Heart Disease Patients," *Psychosomatic Medicine* 61, no. 6 (November–December 1999): 834–841.

2. While medical care for children with congenital heart defects has improved vastly in recent years, relatively little support is available for adults who have such conditions. I have even heard from readers who said they had trouble finding a physician with experience in this specialty. You can get help by contacting the American Heart Association (see Resources, p. 257); if you're connected to the Web, go to www.americanheart.org, click on "Diseases & Conditions," and then click on "Adults with Congenital Heart Disease." You can also visit www.4hcm.org, a site operated by the Hypertrophic Cardiomyopathy Association, and www.cachnet.org, operated jointly by the Canadian Adult Congenital Heart Network and the Toronto Congenital Cardiac Centre for Adults at the University of Toronto (see p. 261).

Chapter 2: The Four Stages of Heart Illness

1. Study appeared in *The New England Journal of Medicine,* as reported in *The Johns Hopkins Medical Letter: Health After 50,* June 2003, 1.

2. Charles Inlander and Steven Findlay, "High-Volume Medical Care Provides Best Results," *USA Today,* July 15, 2002. *The Journal of the American Medical Association* article cited here reported that 24 percent of patients treated by doctors who treated fewer than five myocardial infarction patients annually had died by the end of a year; doctors who treated more than twenty-four MI patients annually had a patient mortality rate of 20 percent.

3. D. J. Magid, B. N. Calonge, J. S. Rumsfeld, et al., "Relation Between Hospital Primary Angioplasty Volume and Mortality for Patients with Acute MI Treated with Primary Angioplasty vs Thrombolytic Therapy," *The Journal of*

NOTES

the American Medical Association 284 (2000): 3131–3138; P. D. McGrath,
D. E. Wennberg, J. D. Dickens, et al., "Relation Between Operator and Hospital Volume and Outcomes Following Percutaneous Coronary Interventions in the Era of the Coronary Stent," *The Journal of the American Medical Association* 284 (2000): 3139–3144.

4. Inlander and Findlay, "High-Volume Medical Care," citing *The New England Journal of Medicine,* April 2002.

5. T. E. Oxman, D. H. Freeman, Jr., and E. D. Manheimer, "Lack of Social Participation or Religious Strength and Comfort as Risk Factors for Death After Cardiac Surgery in the Elderly," *Psychosomatic Medicine* 57 (1995): 5–15.

6. T. Van Elderen, S. Maes, and E. Dusseldorp, "Coping with Coronary Heart Disease: A Longitudinal Study," *Journal of Psychosomatic Research* 47, no. 2 (August 1999): 175–183.

7. J. Levine, S. Warrenburg, R. Kerns, G. E. Schwartz, R. Delaney, et al., "The Role of Denial in Recovery from Coronary Heart Disease," *Psychosomatic Medicine* 49 (1987): 109–117; S. S. Malan, "Psychosocial Adjustment Following MI: Current Views and Nursing Implications," *Journal of Cardiovascular Nursing* 6, no. 4 (1992): 57–70; Van Elderen, Maes, and Dusseldorp, "Coping with Coronary Heart Disease."

8. Van Elderen, Maes, and Dusseldorp, "Coping with Coronary Heart Disease."

9. Each year, 500,000 women in the United States die of cardiovascular illness, compared to 139,300 from lung cancer, breast cancer, and colon cancer combined. (Source: American Heart Association.)

10. S. A. Shumaker and T. R. Smith, "The Politics of Women's Health," *Journal of Social Issues* 50 (1994): 189–202.

11. R. Martin and K. Lemos, "From Heart Attacks to Melanoma: Do Common-Sense Models of Somatization Influence Symptom Interpretation for Female Victims?" *Health Psychology* 21, no. 2 (2002): 25–32.

12. "Prodromal MI Symptoms More Severe in Black Women," Reuters Medical News, April 15, 2002.

13. R. Martin, E. E. I. Gordon, and P. Lounsby, "Gender Disparities in the Attribution of Cardiac-Related Symptoms: Contribution of Common-Sense Models of Illness," *Health Psychology* 17 (1998): 346–357; K. A. Schulman, J. A. Berlin, W. Harless, J. F. Kerner, S. Sistrunk, et al., "The Effect of Race and Sex on Physicians' Recommendations for Cardiac Catheterization," *The New England Journal of Medicine* 340 (1999): 618–626.

14. Ibid.

15. N. C. Chandra, R. C. Ziegelstein, W. J. Rogers, A. J. Tiefenbrunn, J. M. Gore, et al., "Observations of the Treatment of Women in the United States with Myocardial Infarction: A Report from the National Registry of Myocardial Infarction-I," *Archives of Internal Medicine* 158 (1998): 981–988.

NOTES

16. V. L. Roger, S. J. Jacobsen, and P. A. Pellikka, "Gender Differences in Use of Stress Testing and Coronary Heart Disease Mortality: A Population-Based Study in Olmsted County, Minnesota," *Journal of the American College of Cardiology* 32, no. 2 (1998): 345–352.
17. For more on patients' rights and how to manage your medical care, see Angela Perry, medical ed., *American Medical Association Guide to Talking to Your Doctor* (New York: John Wiley & Sons, 2001).
18. J. Daly, D. Elliott, E. Cameron-Traub, Y. Salamonson, P. Davidson, D. Jackson, C. Chin, and V. Wade, "Health Status, Perceptions of Coping, and Social Support Immediately After. Discharge of Survivors of Acute Myocardial Infarction," *American Journal of Critical Care* 9, no. 1 (January 2000): 62–69.
19. Randi Hutter Epstein, "Facing up to Depression After a Bypass," *The New York Times,* November 27, 2001, p. D8.
20. J. S. Leske and S. A. Pelcynski, "Caregiver Satisfaction with Preparation for Discharge in a Decreased-Length-of-Stay Cardiac Surgery Program," *Journal of Cardiovascular Nursing* 14, no. 1 (1999): 35–43.
21. G. Rose, J. Suls, P. Green, P. Lounsbury, and E. Gordon, "Comparison of Adjustment, Activity, and Tangible Support in Men and Women Patients and Their Spouses During the Six Months Post–Myocardial Infarction," *Annals of Behavioral Medicine* 18 (1996): 264–272.
22. R. Allan and S. Scheidt, eds., *Heart and Mind: The Practice of Cardiac Psychology* (Washington, D.C.: American Psychological Association, 1996).
23. G. W. Roach, M. Kanchuger, C. M. Mangano, M. Newman, N. Nussmeier, R. Wolman, A. Aggarwal, K. Marchall, S. H. Graham, and C. Levy, "Adverse Cerebral Outcomes After Coronary Bypass Surgery. Multicenter Study of Perioperative Ischemia Research Group and the Ischemia Research and Education Foundation Investigators," *The New England Journal of Medicine* 335, no. 25 (December 19, 1996): 1857–1863.
24. J. P. Gold, M. E. Charlson, P. Williams-Russo, et al., "Improvement of Outcomes After Coronary Artery Bypass: A Randomized Trial Comparing Intraoperative High Versus Low Mean Arterial Pressure," *The Journal of Thoracic and Cardiovascular Surgery* 110 (1995): 1302–1314.
25. This material and that which follows is taken from S. R. Waldstein and M. F. Elias, eds., *Neuropsychology of Cardiovascular Disease* (Mahwah, N.J.: Lawrence Erlbaum Associates, 2001).
26. R. S. Vasan, M. G. Larson, E. P. Leip, et al. "Assessment of Frequency of Progression to Hypertension in Nonhypertensive Participants in the Framingham Heart Study: A Cohort Study." *Lancet* 358 (2001): 1682–1686. As cited at www.nhlbi.nih.gov/guidelines/hypertension/express.pdf, June 10, 2003.
27. R. S. Vasan, A. Beiser, S. Seshadri, et al. "Residual Lifetime Risk for Developing Hypertension in Middle-aged Women and Men: The Framingham Heart

Study." *The Journal of the American Medical Association* 287 (2002): 1003–1010. As cited at www.nhlbi.nih.gov/guidelines/hypertension/express.pdf, June 10, 2003.

28. A. P. Jabourian, "Cognitive Function, EEG, and Gait Disorders in Cardiac Arrhythmias One Day Before and Eight Days After Pacemaker Implantation," *Annales Médico-Psychologiques* 153 (1995): 89–105.

29. O. E. Havik and J. G. Maeland, "Verbal Denial and Outcome in Myocardial Infarction Patients," *Journal of Psychosomatic Research* 32 (1988): 145–157; G. G. Lloyd and R. M. Cawley, "Distress or Illness? A Study of Psychological Symptoms After Myocardial Infarctions," *The British Journal of Psychiatry* 142 (1983): 120–125.

30. R. B. Case, A. J. Moss, N. Case, M. McDermott, and S. Eberly, "Living Alone After Myocardial Infarction," *The Journal of the American Medical Association* 267, no. 4 (1992): 515–519; R. B. Williams, J. C. Barefoot, and R. M. Califf, "Prognostic Importance of Social and Economic Resources Among Medically Treated Patients with Angiographically Documented Coronary Artery Disease," *The Journal of the American Medical Association* 267 (1992): 520–524.

31. J. Johnston, J. Foulkes, D. W. Johnston, B. Pollard, and H. Gudmundsdottir, "Impact on Patients and Partners of In-Patient and Extended Cardiac Counseling and Rehabilitation: A Controlled Trial," *Psychosomatic Medicine* 61, no. 2 (March–April 1999): 225–233.

32. T. Caulin-Glaser, M. Blum, R. Schmeizl, H. G. Prigerson, B. Zaret, and C. Mazure, "Gender Differences in Referral to Cardiac Rehabilitation Programs After Revascularization," *Journal of Cardiopulmonary Rehabilitation* 21, no. 1 (January–February 2001): 24–30.

33. G. G. Blackburn, J. M. Foody, D. L. Sprecher, E. Park, C. Apperson-Hansen, and F. J. Pashkow, "Cardiac Rehabilitation Participation Patterns in a Large, Tertiary Care Center: Evidence for Selection Bias," *Journal of Cardiopulmonary Rehabilitation* 20, no. 3 (May–June 2000): 189–195.

34. P. A. Ades, "Cardiac Rehabilitation in Older Coronary Patients," *Journal of the American Geriatrics Society* 47 (1999): 98–105.

35. P. A. Ades, M. L. Waldman, E. T. Poehlman, et al., "Exercise Conditioning in Older Coronary Patients: Submaximal Lactate Response and Endurance Capacity," *Circulation* 88 (1993): 572–577.

36. D. R. Seals, J. M. Hagberg, B. F. Hurley, et al., "Endurance Training in Older Men and Women: I. Cardiovascular Response to Exercise," *Journal of Applied Physiology* 57 (1984): 1024–1029.

37. J. G. Warner, P. H. Brubaker, M. S. Ying Zhu, et al., "Long-Term (5-Year) Changes in HDL Cholesterol in Cardiac Rehabilitation Patients: Do Sex Differences Exist?" *Circulation* 92 (1995): 773–777.

38. K. Ishikawa, T. Ohta, J. Zhang, et al., "Influence of Age and Gender on Exer-

cise Training–Induced Blood Pressure Reduction in Systemic Hypertension," *The American Journal of Cardiology* 84 (1999): 192–196; H. Tanaka, M. J. Reiling, and D. R. Seals, "Regular Walking Increases Peak Limb Vasodilatory Capacity of Older Hypertensive Humans: Implications for Arterial Structure," *Journal of Hypertension* 16 (1998): 423–428.

39. Caulin-Glaser et al., "Gender Differences."
40. G. J. Balady, D. Jette, J. Scheer, and J. Downing, "Changes in Exercise Capacity Following Cardiac Rehabilitation in Patients Stratified According to Age and Gender," *Journal of Cardiopulmonary Rehabilitation* 16, no. 1 (January–February 1996): 38–46.
41. L. H. Kushi, R. M. Fee, A. R. Folsom, et al., "Physical Activity and Mortality in Postmenopausal Women," *The Journal of the American Medical Association* 277 (1997): 1287–1292; J. Stessman, Y. Maaravi, R. Hammerman-Rosenberg, et al., "The Effects of Physical Activity on Mortality in the Jerusalem 70-Year-Olds Longitudinal Study," *Journal of the American Geriatrics Society* 48 (2000): 499–504.
42. Coauthor's interview with Kenneth Kambis, Ph.D., altitude physiologist and associate professor of kinesiology, College of William & Mary, Williamsburg, Virginia, September 18, 2002.
43. T. Van Elderen, S. Maes, and E. Dusseldorp, "Coping with Coronary Heart Disease: A Longitudinal Study," *Journal of Psychosomatic Research* 47, no. 2 (August 1999): 175–183.
44. B. M. Psaty, T. D. Koepsell, E. H. Wagner, et al., "The Relative Risk of Incident Coronary Heart Disease Associated with Recently Stopping the Use of Beta-Blockers," *The Journal of the American Medical Association* 263 (1990): 1653–1657.
45. R. P. Byington, "Beta-Blocker Heart Attack Trial: Design, Methods, and Baseline Results. Beta-Blocker Heart Attack Trial Research Group," *Controlled Clinical Trials* 5, no. 4 (1984): 382–437.

Chapter 3: You Can't Do It Alone

1. S. B. Shanefield, "Myocardial Infarction and Patients' Wives," *Psychosomatics* 31 (1990): 138–145.
2. D. K. Moser, K. Dracup, C. Marsden, "Needs of Recovering Cardiac Patients and Their Spouses: Compared Views," *International Journal of Nursing Studies* 30 (1993): 105–114.
3. Shanefield, "Myocardial Infarction and Patients' Wives."
4. D. Cohen, "Primary Care Checklist for Effective Family Management," *Medical Clinics of North America* 78 (1994): 795–809; S. Dickerson, "Cardiac Spouses' Help-Seeking Experiences," *Clinical Nursing Research* 7, no. 1 (1998): 6–24; P. O'Farrell, J. Murray, and S. B. Hotz, "Psychologic Distress

Among Spouses of Patients Undergoing Cardiac Rehabilitation," *Heart & Lung* 29, no. 2 (March–April 2000): 97–104; K. Arefjord, E. Hallaraker, O. E. Havik, and J. G. Maeland, "Life After a Myocardial Infarction—The Wives' Point of View," *Psychological Reports* 83, no. 3, pt. 2 (December 1998): 1203–1216.

5. Adapted from Fredric J. Pashkow and Charlotte Libov, *The Women's Heart Book: The Complete Guide to Keeping Your Heart Healthy* (New York: Hyperion, 2001).

6. J. Suls, P. Green, G. Rose, P. Lounsbury, and E. Gordon, "Hiding Worries from One's Spouse: Associations Between Coping via Protective Buffering and Distress in Male Post–Myocardial Infarction Patients and Their Wives," *Journal of Behavioral Medicine* 20, no. 4 (August 1997): 333–349.

Chapter 4: No-Nonsense Techniques for Managing Your Recovery Team

1. M. C. Morice, P. W. Serruys, E. Sousa, et al., "A Randomized Comparison of a Sirolimus-Eluting Stent with a Standard Stent for Coronary Revascularization," *The New England Journal of Medicine* 346, no. 23 (2002): 1773–1780.

2. D. Ornish, *Love & Survival: The Scientific Basis for the Healing Power of Intimacy* (New York: HarperCollins, 1998); W. M. Sotile, *Heart Illness and Intimacy: How Caring Relationships Aid Recovery* (Baltimore, Md.: Johns Hopkins University Press, 1992).

3. K. Orth-Gomer, S. P. Wamala, M. Horsten, K. Schenck-Gustafsson, N. Schneiderman, and M. A. Mittleman, "Marital Stress Worsens Prognosis in Women with Coronary Heart Disease: The Stockholm Female Coronary Risk Study," *The Journal of the American Medical Association* 284 (2000): 3008–3014.

4. L. G. Russek and G. E. Schwartz, "Perceptions of Parental Caring Predict Health Status in Midlife: A 35-Year Follow-up of the Harvard Mastery of Stress Study," *Psychosomatic Medicine* 59, no. 2 (1997): 144–149.

5. I have adapted these tips from S. Cohen and Edward Lichtenstein, "Partner Behaviors That Support Quitting Smoking," *Journal of Consulting and Clinical Psychology* 58 (1990): 304–309; and K. Ell and C. Dunkel-Schetter, "Social Support and Adjustment to Myocardial Infarction, Angioplasty, and Coronary Artery Bypass Surgery," in *Social Support and Cardiovascular Disease*, ed. S. A. Shumaker and S. M. Czajkowski (New York: Plenum Press, 1994).

6. R. B. Williams, J. C. Barefoot, and R. M. Califf, "Prognostic Importance of Social and Economic Resources Among Medically Treated Patients with Angio-Graphically Documented Coronary Artery Disease," *The Journal of the American Medical Association* 267 (1992): 520–524.

Chapter 5: Embrace Your New Normal and
Cultivate Heart-Healthy Attitudes

1. R. Anda, D. Williamson, D. James, C. Macera, E. Eaker, A. Glassman, and
J. Marks, "Depressed Affect, Hopelessness, and the Risk of Ischemic Heart
Disease in a Cohort of U.S. Adults," *Epidemiology* 4 (1992): 285–294.
2. M. F. Scheier, K. A. Mathews, J. F. Owens, G. J. Magovern, R. C. Lefebvre,
R. A. Abbot, and C. S. Carver, "Dispositional Optimism and Recovery from
Coronary Artery Bypass Surgery: The Beneficial Effects of Physical and Psychological Well-Being," *Journal of Personality and Social Psychology* 57 (1989):
1024–1040.
3. M. D. Boltwood, C. B. Taylor, M. B. Burke, H. Gorgin, and J. Giacomini,
"Anger Report Predicts Coronary Artery Vasomotor Response to Mental
Stress in Atherosclerotic Segments," *American Journal of Cardiology* 72
(1993): 1361–1365.
4. Martin E. P. Seligman, *Learned Optimism* (New York: Simon & Schuster,
1998).
5. "Beyond Cholesterol: A New Clue to Heart Disease," *The Johns Hopkins
Medical Letter: Health After 50*, March 2003.
6. "Predicting Heart Disease: Beyond Cholesterol," *University of California,
Berkeley, Wellness Letter*, March 2003.
7. Adapted from the work of James O. Prochaska, John C. Norcross, and Carlo
C. DiClemente as described in their book *Changing for Good* (New York:
Avon Books, 1994).
8. G. A. Marlatt, "Relapse Prevention: Theoretical," in *Relapse Prevention*, ed.
R. Gordon (New York: Guilford Press, 1985).
9. C. B. Taylor, N. Houston-Miller, J. D. Kilen, and R. F. DeBusk, "Smoking
Cessation After Acute Myocardial Infarction: Effects of a Nurse-Managed
Intervention," *Annals of Internal Medicine* 113, no. 2 (1990): 118–123.
10. L. Rosenberg, J. R. Palmer, and S. Shapiro, "Decline in the Risk of Myocardial Infarction Among Women Who Give Up Smoking," *The New England
Journal of Medicine* 322 (1990): 213–217.
11. American Lung Association Web site: www.lungusa.org/tobacco/smoking_
factsheet99.html (". . . 43 different cancer-causing chemicals;"); also www.
lungusa.org/tobacco/secondhand_factsheet99.html (". . . flares to 4,000.").
12. Statistics on smoking from American Cancer Society and Centers for Disease
Control and Prevention; see also W. M. Sotile, *Psychosocial Interventions for
Cardiopulmonary Patients: A Guide for Health Professionals* (Champaign, Ill.:
Human Kinetics, 1996).

Chapter 6: Learn to Manage Stress and It Won't Hurt You

1. S. Jacobs, R. Friedman, M. Mittleman, M. Maclure, J. Sherwood, H. Benson, and J. E. Muller, for the MI Onset Investigators, "Nine-Fold Increased Risk of Myocardial Infarction Following Psychological Stress Assessed by a Case-Control Study," *Circulation* 86 (suppl. 1) (1992): 198.
2. S. Kobasa, S. Maddi, and R. Kahan, "Hardiness and Health: A Prospective Study," *Journal of Personality and Social Psychology* 31 (1982): 1–11.
3. S. N. Willich, H. Lowel, M. Lewis, R. Arntz, R. Baur, K. Winther, et al., and the TRIMM Study Group, "Association of Wake Time and the Onset of Myocardial Infarction," *Circulation* 84 (suppl. 6) (1991): 62–67.
4. M. A. Mittleman. M. Maclure, G. H. Tofler, J. B. Sherwood, et al., "Triggering of Acute Myocardial Infarction by Heavy Physical Exertion," *The New England Journal of Medicine* 329 (1993): 1677–1683.
5. M. A. Mittleman, M. Maclure, J. B. Sherwood, R. P. Mulry, G. H. Tofler, S. C. Jacobs, R. Friedman, H. Benson, and J. E. Muller, for the Determinants of Myocardial Infarction Onset Study Investigators, "Triggering of Acute Myocardial Infarction Onset by Episodes of Anger," *Circulation* 92 (1995): 1720–1725.
6. L. K. Altman, "Dangerous Heart Rhythms Rose in New York After 9/11," *The New York Times,* November 21, 2002. None of the 200 study participants had a heart attack or died because they all had implanted defibrillators.
7. J. E. Muller, G. H. Tofler, and P. H. Stone, "Circadian Variations and Triggers of Onset of Acute Cardiovascular Disease," *Circulation* 79 (1989): 733–743.
8. Robert Allan and Stephen Scheidt, *Heart and Mind: The Practice of Cardiac Psychology* (Washington, D.C.: American Psychological Association, 1996), p. 85.
9. A. D. Kanner, J. C. Coyne, C. Shaefer, and R. S. Lazarus, "Comparison of Two Modes of Stress Measurement: Daily Hassles and Uplifts Versus Major Life Events," *Journal of Behavioral Medicine* 4 (1981): 1–39.
10. R. J. Larsen, E. Diener, and R. S. Cropanzano, "Cognitive Operations Associated with Individual Differences in Affect Intensity," *Journal of Personality and Social Psychology* 53 (1987): 767–774.
11. J. W. Reich and A. Zatura, "Life Events and Personal Causation: Some Relationships with Satisfaction and Distress," *Journal of Personality and Social Psychology* 41 (1981): 1002–1012.
12. W. J. Kop, "Chronic and Acute Psychological Risk Factors for Clinical Manifestations of Coronary Artery Disease," *Psychosomatic Medicine* 61, no. 4 (July–August 1999): 476–487.
13. D. Pandya, "Psychological Stress, Emotional Behavior and Coronary Heart Disease," *Comprehensive Therapy* 24, no. 5 (May 1998): 265–271.
14. G. H. Tofler, P. H. Stone, M. Maclure, F. Edelman, V. G. Davis, T. Robertson, E. M. Antman, and J. E. Muller, "Analysis of Possible Triggers of Acute

Myocardial Infarction (the MILIS Study)," *The American Journal of Cardiology* 66 (1990): 22–27.

15. The Normative Aging Study found that men who reported two or more anxiety symptoms had nearly twice the risk of fatal coronary heart disease and nearly four times the risk of sudden cardiac death; see I. Kawachi, D. Sparrow, P. Vokonas, and S. Weiss, "Symptoms of Anxiety and Risk of Coronary Heart Disease," *Circulation* 90 (1994): 2225–2229. Also, the Health Professionals Follow-up Study found that men with the highest anxiety levels were 2.45 times more likely to die from coronary heart disease than men who reported no anxiety symptoms; see I. Kawachi, G. A. Colditz, A. Ascherio, E. B. Rimm, E. Giovannucci, M. J. Stampfer, and W. C. Willett, "Prospective Study of Phobic Anxiety and Risk of Coronary Heart Disease in Men," *Circulation* 89 (1994): 1992–1997.

16. L. Wright, "The Type A Behavior Pattern and Coronary Artery Disease," *American Psychologist* 43 (1988): 1–14; D. Pandya, "Psychological Stress, Emotional Behavior and Coronary Heart Disease," *Comprehensive Therapy* 24, no. 5 (May 1998): 265–271.

17. Redford Williams and Virginia Williams, *Lifeskills* (New York: Times Books, 1997).

18. R. Karasek, D. Baker, F. Marxer, A. Ahlbom, and T. Theorell, "Job Decision Latitude, Job Demands and Cardiovascular Disease: A Prospective Study of Swedish Men," *American Journal of Public Health* 71 (1981): 694–705; R. Karasek and T. Theorell, *Healthy Work: Stress, Productivity, and the Reconstruction of Working Life* (New York: Basic Books, 1990).

19. From M. A. Hlatky, L. C. Lam, K. L. Lee, N. E. Clapp-Channing, R. B. Williams, D. B. Pryor, R. M. Califf, and D. M. Mark, "Job Strain and the Prevalence and Outcome of Coronary Artery Disease," *Circulation* 92 (1995): 327–333.

20. A. Appels, P. Hoppener, and P. Mulder, "A Questionnaire to Assess Premonitory Symptoms of Myocardial Infarction," *International Journal of Cardiology* 17 (1987): 15–24; R. van Diest and A. Appels, "Vital Exhaustion and Depression: A Conceptual Study," *Journal of Psychosomatic Research* 35 (1991): 535–544.

21. A. Appels and P. Mulder, "Fatigue and Heart Disease: The Association Between 'Vital Exhaustion' and Past, Present and Future Coronary Heart Disease," *Journal of Psychosomatic Research* 33 (1989): 727–738.

22. W. J. Kop, A. Appels, C. F. Mendes de Leon, H. B. de Swart, and F. W. Bar, "Vital Exhaustion Predicts New Cardiac Events After Successful Coronary Angioplasty," *Psychosomatic Medicine* 56 (1994): 281–287.

23. A. Appels, P. Hoppener, and P. Mulder, "A Questionnaire to Assess Premoni-

tory Symptoms of Myocardial Infarction," *International Journal of Cardiology* 17 (1987): 15–24.

24. Adapted from Robert Ornstein and David Sobel, *Healthy Pleasures* (Reading, Mass.: Addison-Wesley, 1989).

Chapter 7: Deal with Depression

1. Andrew Solomon, *The Noonday Demon: An Atlas of Depression* (New York: Scribner's, 2001).

2. R. M. Carney, "Prevalence of Major Depressive Disorder in Post–Myocardial Infarction Patients," paper presented at the Society of Behavioral Medicine meeting, Chicago, Illinois, March 18, 1990; S. J. Schleifer, M. M. Macari-Hinson, D. A. Coyle, et al., "The Nature and Course of Depression Following Myocardial Infarction," *Archives of Internal Medicine* 149 (1989): 1785–1789.

3. N. Frasure-Smith, F. Lesperance, and M. Talajic, "Depression Following Myocardial Infarction," *The Journal of the American Medical Association* 270 (1993): 1819–1825.

4. J. C. Barefoot and M. Schroll, "Symptoms of Depression, Acute Myocardial Infarction, and Total Mortality in a Community Sample," *Circulation* 93 (1996): 1976–1980; F. Lesperance, N. Frasure-Smith, M. Juneau, and P. Théroux, "Depression and One-Year Prognosis Following Unstable Angina," *Archives of Internal Medicine* 160 (2000): 1354–1360.

5. C. Welin, G. Lappas, and L. Wilhelmsen, "Independent Importance of Psychosocial Factors for Prognosis After Myocardial Infarction," *Journal of Internal Medicine* 247, no. 6 (June 2000): 629–639.

6. S. Wassertheil-Smoller for the SHEP Cooperative Research Group, "Change in Depression as a Precursor of Cardiovascular Events," *Circulation* 89 (1994): 6.

7. J. Abramson, A. Berger, H. M. Krumholz, and V. Vaccarino, "Depression and Risk of Heart Failure Among Older Persons with Isolated Systolic Hypertension," *Archives of Internal Medicine* 161 (2001): 1725–1730.

8. W. Jiang, J. Alexander, E. Christopher, et al., "Relationship of Depression to Increased Risk of Mortality and Rehospitalization in Patients with Congestive Heart Failure," *Archives of Internal Medicine* 161 (2001): 1849–1856.

9. D. E. Bush, R. C. Ziegelstein, M. Tayback, D. Richter, S. Stevens, H. Zahalsky, and J. A. Fauerbach, "Even Minimal Symptoms of Depression Increase Mortality Risk After Acute Myocardial Infarction," *American Journal of Cardiology* 5 (2001): 337–341.

10. "Beyond the Blues: Understanding the Link Between Coronary Artery Disease and Depression," François Lesperance and Allan S. Jaffe, www.medscape.com/viewprogram/1040, February 19, 2002.

11. D. L. Musselman, A. Tomer, A. K. Manatunga, et al., "Exaggerated Platelet Reactivity in Major Depression," *The American Journal of Psychiatry* 153 (1996): 1313–1317.
12. R. M. Carney, K. E. Freedland, M. W. Rich, L. J. Smith, and A. S. Jaffe, "Ventricular Disease and Psychiatric Depression in Patients with Coronary Artery Disease," *The American Journal of Medicine* 95 (1993): 23–28.
13. R. M. Carney, J. A. Blumenthal, P. K. Stein, et al., "Depression, Heart Rate Variability, and Acute Myocardial Infarction," *Circulation* 104 (2001): 2024–2028.
14. P. A. Ades, A. Maloney, P. Savage, et al., "Physical Function in Coronary Patients: Effect of Cardiac Rehabilitation," *Archives of Internal Medicine* 159 (1999): 2357–2360.
15. For an excellent discussion of symptoms of depression, see: J. Preston, *Depression and Anxiety Management* (audiotape) (Oakland, Calif.: New Harbinger Publications, 1992).
16. "Depression: It's More Than Just the Blues," *Johns Hopkins Medical Letter: Health After 50*, May 2003, 3.
17. *Diagnostic and Statistical Manual of Mental Disorders*, 4th ed. (Washington, D.C.: American Psychiatric Association, 1994).
18. E. Goode, M. Peterson, and A. Pollack, "Antidepressants Lift Clouds, but Lose 'Miracle Drug' Label," *The New York Times*, June 30, 2002, p. 1.
19. McFarlane, M. V. Kamath, E. L. Fallen, et al., "Effect of Sertraline on the Recovery Rate of Cardiac Autonomic Function in Depressed Patients After Acute Myocardial Infarction," *American Heart Journal* 142, no. 4 (October 2001): 617–623; V. L. Serebruany, P. A. Gurbel, and C. M. O'Connor, "Platelet Inhibition by Sertraline and N-Desmethylsertraline: A Possible Missing Link Between Depression, Coronary Events, and Mortality Benefits of Selective Serotonin Reuptake Inhibitors," *Pharmacology* 43 (2001): 453–462.
20. I. S. Khawaja and R. E. Feinstein, "Cardiovascular Effects of Selective Serotonin Reuptake Inhibitors and Other Novel Antidepressants." *Heart Disease* 5, no. 2 (2003): 153–160.
21. J. P. Allen, M. J. Eckard, J. Wallen, "Screening for Alcoholism: Techniques and Issues," *Public Health Reports* 103 (1988): 586–592; P. D. Cleary, M. Miller, B. T. Bush, et al., "Prevalence and Recognition of Alcohol Abuse in a Primary Care Population," *The American Journal of Medicine* 86 (1988): 466–471.
22. J. A. Ewing, "Detecting Alcoholism: The CAGE Questionnaire," *The Journal of the American Medical Association* 252 (1984): 1905–1907; R. A. Matano and A. B. Bronstone, "Assessment, Intervention, and Referral of Patients Suffering from Alcoholism," *Journal of Cardiopulmonary Rehabilitation* 14 (1994): 27–29.

23. Ewing, "Detecting Alcoholism."
24. "Depression Study Backs Long Drug Therapy," by the Associated Press, in *The New York Times,* February 21, 2003.
25. C. B. Taylor, J. Sallis, R. Needle, "The Relationship Between Physical Activity and Exercise and Mental Health," *Public Health Report* 100 (1985): 195–201.

Chapter 8: Defuse Your Anger Before It Kills You

1. A. Bierce, *The Devil's Dictionary,* 1906, as cited in *The Wit and Wisdom of the 20th Century,* ed. F. S. Pepper (New York: Peter Bedrick Books, 1987).
2. M. A. Mittleman, M. Maclure, J. B. Sherwood, R. P. Mulry, G. H. Tofler, et al., "Triggering of Acute Myocardial Infarction Onset by Episodes of Anger: Determinants of Myocardial Infarction Onset Study Investigators," *Circulation* 92 (1995): 1720–1725.
3. D. Tice and R. F. Baumeister, "Controlling Anger: Self-Induced Emotional Change," in *Handbook of Mental Control,* vol. 5, ed. D. Wenger and J. Pennebaker (Englewood Cliffs, N.J.: Prentice-Hall, 1993).
4. Meyer Friedman and Diane Ulmer, *Treating Type A Behavior—and Your Heart* (New York: Alfred A. Knopf, 1984).
5. Ibid.
6. Review Panel on Coronary-Prone Behavior and Coronary Heart Disease. "Coronary-Prone Behavior and Coronary Heart Disease: A Critical Review," *Circulation* 63 (1981): 1199–1215.
7. C. E. Thoresen and L. H. Powell, "Type A Behavior Pattern: New Perspectives on Theory, Assessment, and Intervention," *Journal of Consulting and Clinical Psychology* 60 (1992): 595–604.
8. J. C. Barefoot, W. G. Dahlstrom, and R. B. Williams, "Hostility, CHD Incidence and Total Mortality: A 25 Year Follow-up Study of 225 Physicians," *Psychosomatic Medicine* 45 (1983): 59–63; M. A. Chesney, M. H. L. Hecker, and G. W. Black, "Coronary-Prone Components of the Type A Behavior in the WCGS: A New Methodology," in *The Type A Behavior Pattern. Research, Theory and Intervention,* ed. B. K. Houston and C. R. Snyder (New York: John Wiley, 1989); J. E. Williams, C. C. Paton, I. C. Siegler, M. L. Eigenbrodt, F. J. Nieto, and H. A. Tyroler, "Anger Proneness Predicts Coronary Heart Disease Risk: Prospective Analysis from the Atherosclerosis Risk in Communities (ARIC) Study," *Circulation* 101 (2000): 2034–2039.
9. F. H. Gabbay, D. S. Krantz, W. J. Kop, S. M. Hedges, J. Klein, J. S. Gottdiener, and A. Rozanski, "Triggers of Myocardial Ischemia During Daily Life in Patients with Coronary Artery Disease: Physical and Mental Activities, Anger and Smoking," *Journal of the American College of Cardiology* 27 (1996): 585–592.

10. G. Ironsen, C. B. Taylor, M. Boltwood, T. Bartzokis, C. Dennis, M. Chesney, D. Spitzer, and G. M. Segal, "Effects of Anger on Left Ventricular Ejection Fraction in Coronary Disease," *The American Journal of Cardiology* 90 (1992): 281–285.

11. Friedman and Ulmer, *Treating Type A Behavior.*

12. R. Williams and V. Williams, *Anger Kills* (New York: HarperPaperbacks, 1993).

13. As cited earlier, the risk that any one episode of anger will trigger a heart attack is very low. That said, heart patients would do well to remember that "the person who becomes angered an average of four times a day spends eight hours each day at greater than twofold increased risk, which translates into a 76% increased risk over the course of a year." R. Allan and S. Scheidt, eds., *Heart and Mind: The Practice of Cardiac Psychology,* reporting on a personal communication with M. Mittleman, December 22, 1995 (Washington, D.C.: American Psychological Association, 1996).

14. T. W. Smith, "Hostility and Health: Current Status of a Psychosomatic Hypothesis," *Health Psychology* 11, no. 3 (1992): 139–150.

15. C. J. Lavie and R. V. Milani, "Effects of Cardiac Rehabilitation and Exercise Training Programs on Coronary Patients with High Levels of Hostility," *Mayo Clinic Proceedings* 74, no. 10 (October 1999): 959–966.

16. C. Tavris, "On the Wisdom of Counting from One to Ten," *Review of Personal and Social Psychology* 3 (1984): 270–291.

17. Thich Nhat Hanh, *Anger: Wisdom for Cooling the Flames* (Los Angeles: Audio Renaissance, 2001).

18. Matthew McKay, Peter D. Rogers, and Judith McKay, *When Anger Hurts: Quieting the Storm Within* (Oakland, Calif.: New Harbinger Press, 1989).

19. Hanh, *Anger.*

20. R. B. Williams, *The Trusting Heart: Great News About Type A Behavior and Your Heart* (New York: Times Books, 1989); W. M. Sotile, "The Psychological Benefits of Exercising," in *Exercise and the Heart in Health and Disease,* 2d ed., rev. and expanded, ed. R. Shephard and H. Miller (New York: Marcel Dekker, 1999).

21. R. B. Williams, "Coronary-Prone Behaviors, Hostility, and Cardiovascular Health: Implications for Behavioral and Pharmacological Interventions," in *Behavioral Medicine Approaches to Cardiovascular Disease Prevention,* ed. K. Orth-Gomer and N. Schneiderman (Hillsdale, N.J.: Lawrence Erlbaum Associates, 1996).

22. Robert Allan, "Anger Management: A Systemic Program to Reduce Unwanted Anger," paper presented at the Third National Conference of the Psychology of Health, Immunity and Disease, the National Institute for the

Clinical Application of Behavioral Medicine, Orlando, Florida, December 6–11, 1991.

23. H. Weisenger, *Anger at Work* (New York: William Morrow, 1995).
24. Williams and Williams, *Anger Kills.*
25. A. W. Siegman, R. A. Anderson, and T. Berger, "The Angry Voice: Its Effects on the Experience of Anger and Cardiovascular Reactivity," *Psychosomatic Medicine* 52 (1991): 631–643.
26. M. Staver, *21 Ways to Diffuse Anger and Calm People Down* (audiotape) (Boulder, Colo.: CareerTrack, 1997).
27. Lynda H. Powell, "The Hook: A Metaphor for Gaining Control of Emotional Reactivity," in Robert Allan and Stephen Scheidt, eds., *Heart and Mind: The Practice of Cardiac Psychology* (Washington, D.C.: American Psychological Association, 1996), pp. 313–327.
28. Friedman and Ulmer, *Treating Type A Behavior.*

Chapter 9: Reclaim Your Sex Life and Physical Intimacy

1. H. A. Taylor, "Sexual Activity and the Cardiovascular Patient: Guidelines," *The American Journal of Cardiology* 84 (1999): 6N–10N.
2. Ibid.
3. C. Papadopoulos, S. I. Shelley, M. St. Piccolo, C. Beaumont, and L. Barnett, "Sexual Activity After Coronary Bypass Surgery," *Chest* 90 (1986): 681–685.
4. T. Jaarsma, K. Dracup, J. Walden, and L. W. Stevenson, "Sexual Function in Patients with Advanced Heart Failure," *Heart Lung* (July–August, 1996); 25 (4): 262–270.
5. H. Mickley, J. Petersen, and B. L. Nielsen, "Subjective Consequences of Permanent Pacemaker Therapy in Patients Under the Age of Retirement," *PACE (Pacing and Clinical Electrophysiology)* 12 (1989): 401–405.
6. Ibid.; B. Bunzel, G. Wollenek, A. Grundbock, and P. Schramek, "Heart Transplantation and Sexuality: A Study of 62 Male Patients" (in German), *Herz* (1994): 294–301.
7. Sheryl Gay Stolberg, "Pump Extends Lives, and Raises Questions," *The New York Times,* July 2, 2002, p. D1.
8. L. R. Schoer and S. B. Jensen, *Sexuality and Chronic Illness: A Comprehensive Approach* (New York: Guilford Press, 1988). Some male PAD patients say that moving vigorously during sex causes them to lose their erection, but that they can achieve and maintain firm erections if the penis is stimulated and they remain relatively still.
9. Taylor, "Sexual Activity and the Cardiovascular Patient."
10. L. Barclay, "New Approaches to Female Sexual Arousal Disorder," *American Urological Association Annual Meeting: Abstracts,* nos. 105158, 102673, May 25, 2002.

11. L. A. Levine, "Erectile Dysfunction: Causes, Diagnosis and Treatment," *Comprehensive Therapy* 15 (1989): 54–58.
12. Y. Drory, S. Kravetz, V. Florian, and M. Weingarten, "Sexual Activity After First Acute Myocardial Infarction in Middle-Aged Men: Demographic, Psychological and Medical Predictors," *Cardiology* 90 (1998): 207–211.
13. H. A. Feldman, I. Goldstein, D. G. Hatzchristou, R. J. Krane, and J. B. McKinlay, "Impotence and Its Medical and Social Correlates: Results of the Massachusetts Male Aging Study, *The Journal of Urology* 151 (1994): 54–61.
14. C. Papadopoulos, S. I. Shelley, M. St. Piccolo, C. Beaumont, and L. Barnett, "Sexual Activity After Coronary Bypass Surgery," *Chest* 90 (1986): 681–685.
15. J. E. Muller, A. Mittleman, M. Maclure, J. B. Sherwood, and G. H. Tofler, "Triggering Myocardial Infarction by Sexual Activity: Low Absolute Risk and Prevention by Regular Physical Exertion—Determinants of Myocardial Infarction Onset Study Investigators," *The Journal of the American Medical Association* 275 (1996): 1405–1409.
16. K. M. Anderson, P. M. Odell, P. W. Wilson, and W. B. Kannel, "Cardiovascular Disease Risk Profiles," *American Heart Journal* 121 (1993): 293–298.
17. M. A. Mittleman, M. Maclure, J. B. Sherwood, R. P. Mulry, G. H. Tofler, et al., "Triggering of Acute Myocardial Infarction Onset by Episodes of Anger: Determinants of Myocardial Infarction Onset Study Investigators," *Circulation* 92 (1995): 1720–1725.
18. M. A. Mittleman, M. Maclure, G. H. Tofler, J. B. Sherwood, R. J. Goldberg, and J. E. Muller, "Triggering of Acute Myocardial Infarction by Heavy Physical Exertion," *The New England Journal of Medicine* 329 (1993): 1677–1683.
19. Mittleman et al., "Triggering of Acute Myocardial Infarction Onset by Episodes of Anger"; R. DeBusk, "Evaluating the Cardiovascular Tolerance for Sex," *The American Journal of Cardiology* 86 (suppl.) (2000): 51F–56F.
20. G. Jackson, "Erectile Dysfunction and Cardiovascular Disease," *International Journal of Clinical Practice* 53 (1999): 363–368.
21. Mittleman et al., "Triggering of Acute Myocardial Infarction by Heavy Physical Exertion."
22. For these and a wealth of other MET levels, see B. D. Ainsworth, W. L. Haskell, A. S. Leon, et al., "Compendium of Physical Activities: Classification of Energy Costs of Human Physical Activities," *Medicine and Science in Sports and Exercise* 25, no. 1 (January 1993): 71–80.
23. R. DeBusk, "Evaluating the Cardiovascular Tolerance for Sex," *The American Journal of Cardiology* 86 (suppl.) (2000): 51F–56F.
24. J. G. Bohlen, J. P. Held, O. Sanderson, and R. P. Patterson, "Heart Rate, Rate-Pressure Product, and Oxygen Uptake During Four Sexual Activities," *Archives of Internal Medicine* 114 (1984): 1745–1748.
25. DeBusk, "Evaluating the Cardiovascular Tolerance for Sex."

26. H. K. Hellerstein and E. H. Friedman, "Sexual Activity in the Post-Coronary Patient," *Archives of Internal Medicine* 125 (1970): 987–999.
27. R. A. Stein, "The Cardiovascular Response to Sexual Activity," *The American Journal of Cardiology* 86 (suppl.) (2000): 27F–29F.
28. G. Jackson, "Sexual Intercourse and Stable Angina Pectoris," *The American Journal of Cardiology* 86 (suppl.) (2000): 35F–37F.
29. G. Jackson, "Sexual Intercourse and Angina Pectoris," *International Rehabilitation Medicine* 3 (1981): 35–37.
30. S. Mann, M. W. M. Craig, B. Goud, and E. B. Raftery, "Coital Blood Pressure in Hypertensives," (abstract) *Circulation* vol. 3 (suppl. 3) (1980): 111–137.
31. Jackson, "Sexual Intercourse and Stable Angina Pectoris."
32. DeBusk, "Evaluating the Cardiovascular Tolerance for Sex."
33. R. Berkow and Fletcher A. Beers, eds., *The Merck Manual of Medical Information: Home Edition* (West Point, Pa.: Merck & Co., 1997), 685.
34. Ibid., 121.
35. Jackson, "Sexual Intercourse and Stable Angina Pectoris."
36. D. Noonan, "You Still Want Statins with That?," *Newsweek,* July 14, 2003, 48–55.
37. S. Bansal, "Sexual Dysfunction in Hypertensive Men: A Critical Review of the Literature," *Hypertension* 12 (1988): 1–10.
38. R. H. Grimm, G. A. Grandits, R. J. Prineas, et al., "Long-Term Effects on Sexual Function of Five Antihypertensive Drugs and Nutritional Hygienic Treatment in Hypertensive Men and Women: Treatment of Mild Hypertension Study (TOMHS)," *Hypertension* 29 (1997): 8–14.
39. H. Croft, E. Settle, T. Hauser, S. Batey, et al., "A Placebo-Controlled Comparison of the Antidepressant Efficacy and Effects on Sexual Functioning of Sustained-Release Bupropion and Sertraline," *Clinical Therapeutics* 21 (1999): 643–658.
40. R. T. Segraves, H. Croft, R. Kavoussi, et al., "Bupropion Sustained Release (SR) for the Treatment of Hypoactive Sexual Desire Disorder (HSDD) in Non-Depressed Women," *Journal of Sex and Marital Therapy* 27 (2001): 303–316.
41. Merritt McKinney, "Antidepressant Safe After Heart Attack: Study," Reuters; reported on MedlinePlus (www.medlineplus.gov), Web site of the National Library of Medicine.
42. S. P. Roose, G. W. Dalack, A. H. Glassman, et al., "Cardiovascular Effects of Bupropion in Depressed Patients with Heart Disease," *The American Journal of Psychiatry* 148 (1991): 512–516.
43. W. W. Shen, Z. Urosevich, and D. O. Clayton, "Sildenafil in the Treatment of Female Sexual Dysfunction Induced by Selective Serotonin Reuptake

Inhibitors," *The Journal of Reproductive Medicine* 44, no. 6 (June 1999): 535–542.3

44. Barclay, "New Approaches to Female Sexual Arousal Disorder."
45. Harold Silverman, editor-in-chief, *The Pill Book* (New York: Bantam, 2002).
46. C. M. Meston and J. R. Heiman, "Ephedrine-Activated Sexual Arousal in Women," *Archives of General Psychiatry* 55 (1998): 652–656.
47. S. Bent, T. N. Tiedt, M. C. Odden, M. G. Shlipak, "The Relative Safety of Ephedra Compared with Other Herbal Products," *Annals of Internal Medicine* 138 (2003): 468–471.
48. C. A. Haller and N. L. Benowitz, "Adverse Cardiovascular and Central Nervous System Events Associated with Dietary Supplements Containing Ephedra Alkaloids," *The New England Journal of Medicine* 343 (2000): 833–838.
49. M. Herper, "Viagra's Competetion Heats Up," www.forbes.com/2003/04/28/cx_mh_0428viagra_print, April 28, 2003.
50. R. A. Kloner, "Sex and the Patient with Cardiovascular Risk Factors: Focus on Sildenafil," *The American Journal of Cardiology* 109, no. 9A (2000): 13S–21S.
51. C. R. Conti, C. J. Pepine, and M. Sweeney, "Efficacy and Safety of Sildenafil Citrate in Treatment of Erectile Dysfunction in Patients with Ischemic Heart Disease," *The American Journal of Cardiology* 83 (1999): 29C–34C.
52. D. J. Webb, S. Freestone, M. J. Allen, and G. J. Muirhead, "Sildenafil Citrate and Blood-Pressure Lowering Drugs: Results of Drug Interaction Studies with an Organic Nitrate and a Calcium Antagonist," *The American Journal of Cardiology* 83 (suppl.) (1999): 21C–28C.
53. M. D. Chetlin, A. M. Hutter, R. G. Brindis, et al. (ACC/AHA Expert Consensus Document), "Use of Sildenafil (Viagra) in Patients with Cardiovascular Disease," *Journal of the American College of Cardiology* 33 (1999): 273–282.
54. R. A. Kloner, "Cardiovascular Risk and Sildenafil," *The American Journal of Cardiology* 86 (suppl.) (2000): 57F–61F.
55. K. E. Andersson and C. Stief, "Penile Erection and Cardiac Risk: Pathophysiologic and Pharmacologic Mechanisms," *The American Journal of Cardiology* 86 (suppl.) (2000): 23F–26F.
56. Y. Vardi and I. Gruenwald, "Cardiovascular Effects of Oral Pharmacotherapy in ED," *Current Medical Research and Opinion* 16 (suppl. 1) (2000): S43–S47.
57. K. Jones, *Heart Smart Sex: A Guide for Heart Patients and Their Partners* (Charlotte, N.C.: Mecklenburg Cardiac Rehabilitation Center, 1995).

Chapter 10: Believe in Something Greater than Yourself

1. R. A. Hummer, R. G. Rogers, C. B. Nam, and C. G. Ellison, "Religious Involvement and US Adult Mortality," *Demography* 36 (1999): 273–285.

2. F. Luskin, "Review of the Effect of Spiritual and Religious Factors on Mortality and Morbidity with a Focus on Cardiovascular and Pulmonary Disease," *Journal of Cardiopulmonary Rehabilitation* 20 (2000): 8–15.

3. Luskin, "Spiritual and Religious Factors"; D. A. Matthews, H. G. Koenig, C. E. Thoresen, et al., eds., *Scientific Research on Spirituality and Health: A Consensus Report* (Rockville, Md.: National Institute for Healthcare Research, 1998), 31–54.

4. Luskin, "Spiritual and Religious Factors."

5. C. Wallis, "Faith and Healing," *Time*, June 24, 1996, 58–63.

6. Luskin, "Spiritual and Religious Factors"; Matthews et al., eds., *Spirituality and Health*.

7. R. P. Sloan and E. Bagiella, "Claims About Religious Involvement and Health Outcomes," *Annals of Behavioral Medicine* 24, no. 1 (2002): 14–21.

8. C. E. Thoresen and A. H. S. Harris, "Spirituality and Health: What's the Evidence and What's Needed?", *Annals of Behavioral Medicine* 24, no. 1 (2002): 3–13.

9. Ibid.

10. B. J. Zinnbauer, K. I. Pargament, B. Cole, et al., "Religion and Spirituality: Unfuzzying the Fuzzy," *Journal for the Scientific Study of Religion* 36 (1997): 549–564.

11. L. Shahabi, L. H. Powell, M. A. Musick, et al., "Correlates of Self-Perceptions of Spirituality in American Adults," *Annals of Behavioral Medicine* 24, no. 1 (2002): 59–68.

12. L. G. Underwood and J. A. Teresi, "The Daily Spiritual Experience Scale: Development, Theoretical Description, Reliability, Explanatory Factor Analysis, and Preliminary Construct Validity Using Health-Related Data," *Annals of Behavioral Medicine* 24, no. 1 (2000): 22–33; A. H. Peterman, G. Fitchett, M. J. Brady, L. Hernandez, and D. Cella, "Measuring Spiritual Well-Being in People with Cancer: The Functional Assessment of Chronic Illness Therapy—Spiritual Well-Being Scale (FACIT-Sp.)," *Annals of Behavioral Medicine* 24, no. 1 (2002): 49–58; J. L. Shaffer, "Spiritual Distress and Critical Illness," *Critical Care Nurse* 11, no. 1 (1991): 42–45; B. Cortis, *Heart & Soul: A Psychological and Spiritual Guide to Preventing and Healing Heart Disease* (New York: Villard Books, 1995).

13. D. Oman, C. E. Thoresen, and K. McMahon, "Volunteerism and Mortality," *Journal of Health Psychology* 4 (1999): 301–316.

Chapter 11: Living Well with Heart Failure (HF)

1. Marc Silver, *Success with Heart Failure Revised* (Cambridge, Mass.: Perseus Publishing, 2002).
2. Ibid.
3. G. Kolata, "2 Altered Genes Are Linked To Congestive Heart Failure," *The New York Times,* October 10, 2002.
4. L. K. Altman, "Follow-Up Calls Aid Heart-Failure Cases," *The New York Times,* November 19, 2002.
5. Kolata, "2 Altered Genes."
6. D. Levy, S. Kenchaiah, M. G., Larson, et al., "Long-Term Trends in the Incidence of and Survival with Heart Failure," *The New England Journal of Medicine* 347 (2002): 1397–1402.
7. "Congestive Heart Failure in the United States: A New Epidemic," www.nhlbi.nih.gov/health/public/heart/other/CHF.pdf (accessed October 21, 2002).
8. D. R. Moser and P. L. Worster, "Effect of Psychosocial Factors on Physiologic Outcomes in Patients with Heart Failure," *Journal of Cardiovascular Nursing* 14, no. 4 (2000): 106–115.
9. J. C. Coyne, M. Rohrbaugh, J. Shoham, S. Sonnega, J. Nicklas, and J. Cranford, "Prognostic Importance of Marital Quality for Survival of Congestive Heart Failure," *The American Journal of Cardiology* 88 (2001): 526–529.
10. Silver, *Success with Heart Failure.*
11. H. M. Krumholz, J. Butler, J. Miller, et al., "Prognostic Importance of Emotional Support for Elderly Patients Hospitalized with Heart Failure," *Circulation* 97 (1998): 958–964.
12. T. A. Murberg and E. Bru, "Social Relationships and Mortality in Patients with Congestive Heart Failure," *Journal of Psychosomatic Research* 5, no. 1 (September 2001): 521–527.
13. "Congestive Heart Failure: How Can I Follow a Low-Salt Diet?," www.heartpoint.com/congheartfailuretellme.html (accessed October 28, 2002).
14. J. B. Conti, "Bi-Ventricular Pacing Therapy for Congestive Heart Failure: A Review of the Literature," *Cardiology Review* 9 (2001): 217–226.
15. W. T. Abraham, W. G. Fisher, A. L. Smith, et al., "The MIRACLE Study Group: Cardiac Resynchronization in Chronic Heart Failure," *The New England Journal of Medicine* 346 (2002): 1845–1853.
16. R. N. Fogoros, "New Heart Failure Treatment Continues to Impress," www.heartdisease.about.com/library/weekly/aa061402a.htm, June 14, 2002.
17. Ibid.
18. D. Grady, "When Her Heart Failed, a Pump Gave Her Life," *The New York Times,* June 10, 2003.

Chapter 12: Living Well with an Implantable Cardioverter Defibrillator (ICD)

1. Deborah Daw Heffernan, *An Arrow Through the Heart: One Woman's Story of Life, Love, and Surviving a Near-Fatal Heart Attack* (New York: Free Press, 2002).

2. A. J. Moss, W. Zareba, W. J. Hall, H. Klein, et al., "Prophylactic Implantation of a Defibrillator in Patients with Myocardial Infarction and Reduced Ejection Fraction," *The New England Journal of Medicine* 346 (2002): 877–882.

3. G. Kolata, "Extending Life, Defibrillators Can Prolong Misery," *The New York Times,* March 25, 2002.

4. S. C. Vlay, L. C. Olson, G. L. Fricchione, and R. Friedman, "Anxiety and Anger in Patients with Ventricular Tachyarrhythmias: Responses After Automatic Internal Cardioverter Defibrillator Implantation," *PACE (Pacing and Clinical Electrophysiology)* 12 (1989): 366–373; S. F. Sears, A. E. Eads, S. Marhefka, W. M. Sotile, et al., "The U.S. National Survey of Implantable Cardioverter Defibrillator Recipients: Examining the Global and Specific Aspects of Quality of Life," abstract presented to the 21st Congress of the European Society of Cardiology, Barcelona, Spain, August 28–September 1, 1999.

5. A. J. Moss, D. Cannom, et al., for the Multicenter Automatic Defibrillator Implantation Trial (MADIT), "Improved Survival with an Implanted Defibrillator in Patients with Coronary Disease at High Risk for Ventricular Arrhythmia," *The New England Journal of Medicine* 335 (1996): 1933–1940.

6. J. S. Steinberg, J. B. Martins, M. Domanski, et al., "Antiarrhythmic Drug Use in the Implantable Defibrillator Arm of the Antiarrhythmics Versus Implantable Defibrillators (AVID) Study," *Journal of the American College of Cardiology* 31 (1998): 514A.

7. A. J. Moss, W. Zareba, J. Hall, H. Klein, D. J. Wilber, D. S. Cannom, J. P. Daubert, S. L. Higgins, M. W. Brown, and M. L. Andrews, for *The New England Journal of Medicine,* "Prophylactic Implantation of a Defibrillator in Patients with Myocardial Infarction and Reduced Ejection Fraction," *The New England Journal of Medicine* 346, no. 12 (2002): 877–881.

8. Altman, "Dangerous Heart Rhythms Rose in New York After 9/11."

9. Sears et al., "U.S. National Survey."

10. For information on the Stanford Cellular Technology Study, see the summary of proceedings of the May 2002 conference of the North American Society of Pacing and Electrophysiology (PACE) at www.naspe.org.

11. B. W. Ramo, "Ask the Doctor: Protecting Cheney's Heart," *Health Update,* January 2002, 20–21.

12. J. L. Jones, "Ventricular Fibrillation." In: I. Singer, ed., *Implantable Cardioverter Defibrillator* (Armonk, N.Y.: Futura Publishing, 1994).

13. S. F. Sears, J. F. Todaro, T. S. Lewis, W. M. Sotile, and J. B. Conti, "Examining the Psychosocial Impact of Implantable Cardioverter Defibrillators: A Literature Review," *Clinical Cardiology* 28 (1999): 481–489.

14. C. M. Dougherty, "Psychological Reactions and Family Adjustment in Shock Versus No Shock Groups After Implantation of Internal Cardioverter Defibrillator," *Heart & Lung* 24 (1995): 281–291.

15. R. O. Roine, S. Kajaste, and M. Kaste, "Neuropsychological Sequelae of Cardiac Arrest," *The Journal of the American Medical Association* 269 (1993): 237–242; M. J. Sauve, J. A. Walker, S. M. Massa, et al., "Patterns of Cognitive Recovery in Sudden Cardiac Arrest Survivors: The Pilot Study," *Heart & Lung* 25 (1996): 172–181.

16. E. Bass, "Cardiopulmonary Arrest: Pathophysiology and Neurologic Complications," *Annals of Internal Medicine* 103, no. 6 (1985): 920–997; J. J. Carrona and S. Finkelstein, "Neurological Syndrome After Cardiac Arrest," *Current Concepts in Cerebrovascular Disease* 13 (1978): 9–14.

17. C. M. Dougherty, "The Natural History of Recovery Following Sudden Cardiac Arrest and Internal Cardioverter-Defibrillator Implantation," *Progress in Cardiovascular Nursing* 16, no. 4 (2001): 163–168.

18. Sears et al., "Examining the Psychosocial Impact."

19. R. L. Wallace, S. F. Sears, T. S. Lewis, J. T. Griffis, et al., "Predictors of Quality of Life in Long-Term Recipients of Implantable Cardioverter Defibrillators," *Journal of Cardiopulmonary Rehabilitation* 22, no. 4 (2002): 278–281.

20. S. M. Bremner, K. M. McCauley, and K. A. Axtell, "A Follow-up Study of Patients with Implantable Cardioverter Defibrillators," *Journal of Cardiovascular Nursing* 7, no. 3 (1993): 40–51.

21. Ibid.

22. Sandeep Jauhar, "Jolts of Anxiety," *The New York Times,* May 5, 2002.

23. Dougherty, "Psychological Reactions and Family Adjustment."

24. W. M. Sotile and S. F. Sears, *You Can Make a Difference: Brief Psychosocial Interventions for ICD Patients and Their Families* (Minneapolis, Minn.: Medtronic, 1999).

25. Bremner et al., "A Follow-up Study."

26. Heffernan, *An Arrow Through the Heart.*

27. E. White, "Patients with Implantable Cardioverter Defibrillators: Transition to Home," *Journal of Cardiovascular Nursing* 14, no. 3 (2000): 42–52.

28. For more information on electromagnetic interference and how it can affect your ICD, see Medtronic's Web site: medtronic.com/rhythms/downloads/icd_en199300962cEN.pdf.

29. J. M. Craney and M. T. Powers, "Factors Related to Driving in Persons with

an Implantable Cardioverter Defibrillator," *Progressive Cardiovascular Nursing* 10, no. 3 (1995): 12–17; N. Finch, R. Leman, J. Drantz, et al., "Driving Safety Among Patients with Automatic Implantable Cardioverter Defibrillators," *The Journal of the American Medical Association* 270 (1993): 1587–1588.

30. W. Jung and B. Luderitz, "Quality of Life and Driving in Recipients of the Implantable Cardioverter-Defibrillator," *The American Journal of Cardiology* 8, no. 5A (1996): 51–56.

31. Ibid.

32. C. R. Chapman and D. Morrison, "Impacts on Earth by Asteroids and Comets: Assessing the Hazard," *Nature* 367 (1994): 33–40. As reported on the Web site of the California State University at San Bernardino, geology. csusb.edu/360/chnc&die.htm (accessed October 21, 2002).

33. R. Wallace, K. Campbell, R. Sotile, S. F. Sears, et al., "Women and the Implantable Cardioverter Defibrillator: A Lifespan Perspective," *Clinical Cardiology*, in press. Also see A. Natale, T. Davidson, M. J. Geiger, and K. Newby, "Implantable Cardioverter-Defibrillators and Pregnancy: A Safe Combination?," *Circulation* 96, no. 9 (1997): 2808–2812.

Appendix

1. D. W. Sifton, editor in chief, *The PDR Pocket Guide to Prescription Drugs*, 5th ed. (New York: Pocket Books, 2002); H. M. Silverman, editor in chief, *The Pill Book* (New York: Bantam Books, 2002); R. Allan and S. Scheidt, eds., *Heart and Mind: The Practice of Cardiac Psychology* (Washington, D.C.: American Psychological Association, 1996); F. J. Pashkow and C. Libov, *The Women's Heart Book: The Complete Guide to Keeping Your Heart Healthy* (New York: Hyperion, 2001); F. J. Pashkow and W. A. Dafoe, eds., *Clinical Cardiac Rehabilitation: A Cardiologist's Guide*, 2d ed. (Baltimore: Williams & Wilkins, 1999).

2. Merritt McKinney, "Antidepressant Safe After Heart Attack: Study," Reuters Health, August 13, 2002, originally reported in *The Journal of the American Medical Association* 288 (2002): 701–709, 750–751.

3. L. K. Altman, "2 Studies Point to Altered Approach on Atrial Fibrillation," *The New York Times*, December 5, 2002.

4. Ibid.

INDEX

depression (*cont.*)
  counseling for, 44, 129, 132
  as curable, 117
  dangers of, 115–16
  epidemic of, 114
  exercise for, 117, 130
  grief, as compared to, 128
  heart health affected by, 116–17
  in homecoming, 18–19, 30–31
  identification of, 118–19
  imagine it, act it, become it
    technique for, 129–30
  instant gratification as temporary
    relief for, 124–25
  medical help for, 121–27
  negative thinking in, 68–69
  and physical functioning, 117,
    120
  planning your schedule to
    alleviate, 130–31
  relationships require attention in
    cases of, 131–32
  signs of, 119–21
  and stress, 93
  as symptom of something else,
    122, 128–29
  thinking, 119–20, 127–29
  tips for dealing with, 132–33
  vital exhaustion compared to,
    98
despair, 27; *see also* depression
diaphragmatic breathing, 106
diary, keeping journal or, 144–45
diastole, 200
diastolic dysfunction, 200
diet:
  and depression, 120
  and health, 111
  resources, 260
  salt in, 207–8

dietary supplements, cholesterol-
    lowering, 253
digitalis, 212
digoxin, 212
disappointment, overreacting to,
    192
disorientation, 28
diuretics, 212, 246
doctors, *see* physicians
dopamine reuptake inhibitors,
    243
dreams, disturbing, 29
driving, with an ICD, 235–36
drugs, *see* medication
Durable Power of Attorney for
    Health Care, 194
duties and obligations, 129
dynamic cardiomyoplasty, 217

ejection fraction, 166, 223
electrical shocks, with an ICD, 224,
    227–29, 232, 234
electrolytes, 212
electromagnetic interference (EMI),
    234, 235
emotions:
  behind the message, 61
  coping with, 34, 204–11
  in grief, 27
  identification of, 12
  mood changes, 28
  numbness vs., 108
  posttraumatic stress disorder, 21,
    27–31
  sex and, 179
  surging, 15
  talking about, 35, 146
encouragement, 34
energy, soulful, 204
entertainment, reading for, 111

guilt (*cont.*)
  and homecoming, 27
  New Age, 74

hallucinations, 28
happiness, 111, 193
harmony, 193
Harold (focus on bottom line), 73
healing, and religion, 188, 189
heart attack:
  and cognitive functioning, 23
  depression and, 115
  risk profile for, 164–67
  sex and, 156, 160, 174
  signs and symptoms of, 45
  stress and, 89
  surviving, 10
  see also myocardial infarction (MI)
heart disease:
  denial of, 11–14
  depression and, 116–17
  learning about, 31
  passive acceptance of, 49
  resources, 257–58
  risk factors of, 89–90
  risk profiles for, 165–67
  stage 1: survival, 8–15
  stage 2: coping, 15–18
  stage 3: homecoming, 17–31
  stage 4: living with the disease, 29–36
  symptoms and signs of, 45–46
  thinking about, 70
  wait-and-see period in, 9
  women and, 13–14
heart failure (HF), 197–218
  achievement vs. expectation, 203–4
  active management of, 198
  chronic, 25
  classes of, 202

clinics, 203
and cognitive functioning, 24
coping with, 202–3
and exercise, 209–11
genetics and, 197
information gathering in, 213–18
left-sided, 200–201
managing life with, 204–11
and medications, 208, 211–13
right-sided, 201–3
risk factors, 198
and sex, 157
and stress, 206
symptoms of, 201–2, 217–18
as syndrome, 199
use of term, 199–200
when to call the doctor, 217–18
heart-healthy living:
  adjustments to, 31–36, 67–68, 205–6
  behavior changes in, 74–86
  control in, 33
  diet, 111, 260
  exercise, 76
  family relationships in, 76; *see also* families
  first goals for, 32–34
  healing, 189
  imagine it, act it, become it technique, 76, 129–30
  individual pace of change in, 57–58
  information about, 31, 57
  process of changing behaviors, 74–75
  sedentary, dangers of being, 166, 175
  smoking, 85–86, 111, 207, 260
  stages of change in, 79–85
  stress management, 77–78
  thinking patterns, 67–68

Permissions

ABOUT THE AUTHORS

Wayne M. Sotile, Ph.D.
Since 1979, Wayne M. Sotile, a clinical psychologist, has served as Director of Psychological Services at the Wake Forest University Cardiac Rehabilitation Program. With his wife, Mary O. Sotile, he is codirector of Sotile Psychological Associates and Real Talk, Inc., in Winston-Salem, North Carolina.

A pioneer in bringing family systems concepts into the treatment of cardiac patients, Dr. Sotile is a Fellow of the American Association for Cardiovascular and Pulmonary Rehabilitation (AACVPR), an Approved Supervisor in the American Association for Marriage and Family Therapy, and an Honorary Fellow in the American Academy of Medical Administrators.

Dr. Sotile serves on the editorial advisory boards of several leading professional journals and is an expert on physician well-being; he and Mary O. Sotile serve as managing editors of *The Resilient Physician Newsletter.* Dr. Sotile's work is often featured on national television and in international print and radio media.

Dr. Sotile travels throughout the world as a keynote speaker, teaching communities, businesses, professional organizations, and heart patients and their families how to cultivate resilience and thrive with heart disease.

Wayne M. Sotile, Ph.D.
1396 Old Mill Circle
Winston-Salem, North Carolina 27103
Telephone: (336) 765-3032
Fax: (336) 760-6977
E-mail: realtalk@triad.rr.com
Web sites: www.sotile.com
       www.ThrivingWithHeartDisease.com

Robin Cantor-Cooke
Robin Cantor-Cooke has worked extensively in the self-help field as a writer, editor, and audio scriptwriter and producer on more than forty books and tape programs. She has a master's degree from the Medill School of Journalism, Northwestern University, and lives in Williamsburg, Virginia. You may reach her at robcancook@cox.net.

LaVergne, TN USA
10 June 2010
185645LV00001B/67/P